MW01087807

Dr. Jo's
Fit in 15
Minutes per Week

BESSIE JO TILLMAN, MD
P.J. TILLMAN

Copyright (c) 2015 Bessie Jo and Pat Tillman
All rights reserved.
ISBN-10: 1511619376
ISBN-13: 978-1511619370

DEDICATION

Dedicated to you! We dedicate this book to everyone who ever wanted to start an exercise program but didn't quite know where to start or what the best program would be. May you enjoy success and realize optimal health as you embark on this adventure.

We also dedicate this book to you if you have exercised faithfully for years and now you're ready for an amazing program that keeps you optimally fit and frees up a lot of time that you previously devoted to exercise. Enjoy your new found freedom.

TABLE OF CONTENTS

ACKNOWLEDGMENTS

Here we say thank you to some special people who generously contributed to the production of this book. We so appreciate our models who demonstrated the proper weight lifting forms for the photos, our wonderful grandson Andrew Nail and our dear friend and good sport Cathy Blevins. A big thank you also to our friend and photographer Heather Sherman for all of her patience and expertise in photographing the pictures for this book.

RESOURCES

Resources for your Fit in 15 workouts:

http://www.drjomd.com/products/fit-in-15-minutes-per-week/

Workout logs to record your progress

http://www.drjomd.com/products/fit-in-fifteen-workout-logs/

More Fit in 15 information

http://www.drjomd.com/fit-in-15-minutes-per-week/

Dr. Jo's web site

www.drjomd.com

More products by Dr. Jo

http://www.drjomd.com/products/

CHAPTER 1
HISTORY OF FIT IN 15

What If All of This Could Happen to You with Just 15 Minutes of <u>Effort per Week</u>?

- Could This Be True? In just 15 minutes per week you could:
- Increase your glucose storage capacity (help reverse Type 2 diabetes)
- Increase your muscle mass
- Lose fat faster
- Strengthen your heart, even after a heart attack
- Increase your lung volume
- Raise HDL cholesterol (the "good guy")
- Add years of healthy living to your life
- Boost your immune system

It's got to be hype! I know that was my first response to hearing that all of those wondrous results in transforming my body to a high level of fitness could occur with only 15 minutes per week of effort. It does sound absolutely unbelievable.

But do you know what? It's true and it's not such a new concept. But if it's been around for such a long time why didn't I know about it sooner? Probably because there just hasn't been much media attention to it. So it's been very much underutilized. That left me and maybe you also stuck in the old paradigm.

Back in the early 1980's when I first became interested in wellness and prevention of disease I travelled to Dallas, Texas to Dr. Cooper's Aerobics Clinic to participate in a seminar on exercise and how to measure fitness levels. It was a great course and even introduced me to healthy nutrition.

Dr. Cooper brought the benefits of exercise into the public awareness and published his book in 1968. My copy is still sitting on my book shelf. He helped a lot of people improve their health. His exercise physiology research center scientifically measured the healthy improvements in the physiology of folks who participated in various exercise programs for many years.

Dr. Cooper followed many athletes who participated in the long endurance exercises like running and biking, those who did marathons and Iron Man events.

In these endurance exercises, the long slow type, you never have to stop and "catch your breath". I remember the adage, run just fast enough to still be able to talk. This type of exercise creates endurance and efficiency, but something else was happening that was not healthy.

By the late 1980-90s Dr. Cooper realized that these types of slower, more prolonged exercise were causing more harm than good. People were dropping dead of heart attacks and getting cancer more frequently than the general public.

What went wrong?

Dr. Cooper continued to look at those problems and revised his recommendations. Then along came Dr. Al Sears with new research.

Dr. Sears expected long distance runners to have a large lung capacity. Was he ever surprised when he discovered that they had smaller lung capacity.

They also had less muscle mass. Just look at their physique. Most long distance runners have lean, slim bodies.

Dr. Sears also found that their tissues were assaulted with more free radical damage and that they had greater risk of joint or other injury from overuse.

Why was this so?

According to Dr. Doug McGuff, MD (more about him later) endurance exercise is not natural. Watch children and animals. They run seconds to a minute or two. Then stop and plop down or investigate whatever attracts their attention at the moment.

Just try to go on a walk with a kid or a dog-or both. They are definitely not goal oriented and you feel like you will never get to your destination.

Turns out that we should take a lesson from the kids and animals because steady state (endurance) exercise trains plasticity out of your system. It makes you less adaptable. This connotation of plasticity means ability to adapt. Long endurance exercise causes "shrinkage:" smaller muscles, smaller heart and smaller lungs. What's worse, it wipes out your heart's and lung's *reserve capacity.*

Your heart and lungs use their reserve capacity to deal with stress. When faced with a threatening situation where you may need to run or fight:

- Your heart has the ability to pump more blood.
- Your lungs can move more air to increase oxygenation.
- You can deal better with lifting, going upstairs or running.

Seems odd that long distance running or other endurance type of exercises actually decreases your heart's ability to pump blood fast in a threatening situation where you need to sprint, but that's what the current research reveals.

Extreme athletes with their strong determination push themselves and their hearts to the stress point when they run 50 miles or more, repeat marathons too frequently or participate in other extreme sports activities like Ironman Triathlons and very long distance bicycle races. Driving their hearts in this repeated stress mode may cause heart damage.

After athletes complete an extreme running event their blood contains markers associated with heart damage. If the athlete rests enough between events their bodies eliminate these markers within a week. But if they stress their hearts too frequently their hearts may develop thicker heart walls or scars that then decrease the amount of blood the heart can pump with each contraction.[1]

With these changes in the heart anatomy they also increase their risk for heart rhythm problems, especially in a small percentage who have an enlarged heart before they start this extreme sport activity or if they have hardening of the heart arteries. [2]

Most of us have no desire to push ourselves that hard so our moderate forms of exercise actually strengthen the heart. Now we can keep our hearts functioning well in just 15 minutes per week by engaging in the right kind of exercise.

Isn't it just terrific to know that we can keep our hearts, lungs, muscles and the rest of our bodies fit in such a short amount of time? Now we have no room for excuses not to engage in this health promoting exercise form.

That time-efficient, high-fitness-level exercise involves High Intensity Training and specifically the SuperSlow™ technique of strengthening your muscles. In SuperSlow™ exercise participants lift a weight slowly through the range of motion, about 10 seconds up and 10 seconds down using superb form.

Many writers attribute the birth of SuperSlow™ to Ken Hutchins subsequent to his involvement with a study on osteoporosis. He was asked to devise a weight lifting program to strengthen the muscles of ladies with thin bones, pain and weak muscles.

Indeed Mr. Hutchins did research, develop, write and teach about this method extensively and also registered the Trademark SuperSlow™. So crediting him with originating SuperSlow™ can be legitimate.

However, others advocated the slow method of weight lifting as far back as 1895 and perhaps even back to ancient historical times with the Romans, Greeks and Egyptians. In 1895 Dr. John Harvey Kellogg, that physician who advocated healthy lifestyle measures even then, wrote about slowly lifting the weight over 8 seconds and paying attention to good form. (Although he had good intentions, too bad he developed Kellogg's Corn flakes, a not so good carbohydrate.)

In the 1920s Bob Hoffman taught slow weight lifting with proper form as a way to prevent injury when lifting and improve health. Various advocates of slow weight lifting came along after Bob Hoffman.

Perhaps the most influential one was Arthur Jones who in the 1960s developed the Nautilus weight lifting machines and wrote the *Nautilus Protocol.* In 1970 Dr. Bocchiccio, MD suggested to Arthur that using the longer weight lifting time of slowly lifting the weight up for 10 seconds and then slowly moving it down for 10 seconds would improve the results, but neither Arthur nor others accepted that suggestion at that time.

However, about the same time in the early 1970's Jones hired Dr. Ellington Darden to write about Jones' Nautilus program and spread the word. And that he did in great measure by writing volumes of material. In that process he added his refinements to the program.

With the volume of written material he was producing Dr. Darden needed a research assistant. So Jones' magnetic personality attracted Ken Hutchins for the job. And that's how Ken Hutchins eventually became involved in the Nautilus Osteoporosis Project, funded by the Nautilus Company. [3]

Out of concern for his patients who had osteoporosis a doctor at the University of Florida in Gainesville invited Hutchins to set up a muscle strength training program for these fragile women. He theorized that strengthening their back muscles would help alleviate their pain. The project was delayed until Hutchins could solve a significant problem.

"How can older women safely perform exercises on a Nautilus-type machine? Even though these machines are designed for safety we were concerned that our subjects' bones were too brittle to stand up to hard work. We hoped to reverse bone loss, not injure people."[4]

At that time the Nautilus coaches were instructing people to lift the weight in two seconds and return the weight in 4 seconds. But that two second acceleration requires a sudden movement that could be dangerous in folks with thin brittle bones.

The SuperSlow™ concept was conceived when they came up with a solution; use a ten-second very slow exertion with lighter weights. Now the project designers felt comfortable with the safety of the exercise protocol, but would it provide the benefits they were hoping for?

Ultimately the benefits proved to be even better than they had hoped for. From 1982 to 1985 osteoporotic women participated in 6-week or 10-week weight lifting programs using the slow lifting concept with the amazing results of an average of 30% increase in muscle strength in 85 women. They increased their strength even faster than younger people who exercised more vigorously.

Such success motivated Ken Hutchins to delve further into the exercise world. He designed exercise equipment, provided detailed information about that exercise equipment and educated many people about the correct exercise techniques to gain optimal fitness.

Because of his meticulous research and knowledge we should pay close attention to his recommendations about this form of exercise that will benefit us the most in the shortest amount of time.

I honor him and the others that have contributed to the knowledge of the SuperSlow™ program that greatly improves our fitness and health. These researchers have looked intricately into the physiological improvements that the SuperSlow™ weight lifting method makes in our muscles and other organs and the detailed biochemical beneficial changes inside our cells. Although fascinating, some of this scientific information can be overwhelming.

So my desire is to share this information with you in an exciting and understandable way and give you a burning desire to be fit and healthy in only 15 minutes per week! You can do it! And you will love the benefits.

CHAPTER 2
MY INTRODUCTION to
SUPERSLOW™

A quick note—when the author writes in the first person (I) it's Dr. Jo except in the section where Pat tells about his initial encounter with SuperSlow™. "We" refers to Pat and Dr. Jo.

Before discovering SuperSlow™ I had been competing in sprint triathlons, one per year for 15 years. Just before my first grandchild was born at age 53 I crossed the finish line of my first competition! Despite being the last one across the line out of a couple of hundred people I felt a great sense of accomplishment. Simply covering all of that distance (swim about ½ mile, bike 10 miles and run 4.5 miles) fulfilled my goal.

In the following two or three years I came in last a few more times and received the "Tail End Charlie" prize! Then amazingly in subsequent years a number of other folks crossed the finish line after me. I even received a medal in my age group most years. To be honest though there were not a lot of participants in my age group by then (50 and 60 year old women).

Training for these events kept me exercising all year with greater time and effort expended in the two months or so before the triathlon event on the Sunday before Labor Day. The triathlon was my motivation to stay in shape all year. And it was "an event", a gathering, a time to have fun and test your tenacity in a beautiful setting, swimming in a mountain lake, biking in a gorgeous forest and running with views of the forest and a stunning mountain.

But the training was quite time consuming, usually 1.5-2 hours 3 times per week and even more in the two months before the triathlon. Strength training with weights was part of the regimen at least once or twice per week. Fatigue set in the day of the long workouts, biking for 60 minutes, then running for about 70 minutes. I thanked the Lord regularly for my healthy joints but towards the end of my triathlon days one knee was beginning to speak to me a bit. But I was staying in great shape!

Or so I thought!

Then I watched Dr. Mercola interview Dr. McGuff about the SuperSlow™ concept and my brain lit up! You mean I can exercise once per week for 15 minutes and get better results than spending 6 to 9 hours per week in training? Wow, that would free up a lot of time! I really like that idea.

And I can avoid joint injury and other wear and tear on the body! That means I can stay healthier and be fit at the same time because of less possibility of injury. Sounds very good to me!

It occurred to me that I had been overtraining. When there's a better way let's do it the better way.

Dr. McGuff's SuperSlow™ program intrigued me. By profession he's an emergency room physician but he's been interested in exercise since his days of BMX racing at age 14. That interest turned to studying exercise and working with everyday folks in his fitness programs for the last 11 years. In his studies he discovered the physiology behind the success of high intensity training.

Before you start thinking, "I cannot do this program," hear what Dr. McGuff says. **Anyone Can Do His Program.** The oldest they've had in the program was 93, and they have folks in their 80's now. For you see this program adapts to your level of fitness when you enter the program. You simply start by finding your current level of capabilities. Then ask 100 % of those capabilities at the moment. You have a built in safety switch. Your own condition will prevent you from overstressing yourself.

Remember the birth of SuperSlow™, it all started when Ken Hutchins developed the slow weight lifting program for the ladies with osteoporosis. They had brittle bones and weak muscles but their strength improved an average of 30% in six to eight weeks of the SuperSlow™ workouts. If they can do it almost anyone can participate.

But of course you must always check with your physician before embarking on an exercise program especially if you are over 40 years old and/or have not been physically active. Also, anyone with an injury must be supervised by a professional during a slow weight training program. The method of lifting may need to be modified to accommodate the injury.

My husband's first response to the SuperSlow™ concept

My husband Pat enjoys exercise. He loves to participate in it, to promote it and loves the benefits of exercising. He pays great attention to the details of proper lifting of weights or proper training in a sport like bicycling or playing basketball or tennis. His scientific mind creates forms to record the exercise gains.

From the time following our marriage he led the way in keeping our family healthy through exercise. When coaching others he explains procedures very clearly and coaches in a remarkably encouraging way.

For years he studied weight lifting techniques following the gurus in that field. He also spent hours at the gym or in our home lifting weights, sometimes for two hours three times per week.

So in my excitement of discovering the SuperSlow™ technique of muscle strengthening I shared my enthusiasm with him. At that point he didn't reveal his initial skepticism to me and graciously took it under consideration. Later he shared this:

ONE MAN'S EXPERIENCE WITH SUPER SLOW WEIGHT TRAINING—by Pat Tillman

Weightlifting has been an important part of my life and wellbeing for over 50 years, having started in my early twenties. During that time I've experimented with many different programs, read a number of books on the subject of weightlifting and worked with many outstanding trainers— and some who were not so outstanding. I have trained or helped train other lifters on safe and efficient lifting methods. I have had my share of successes and difficulties.

I became aware of high intensity training, using the super slow method, about three years ago. My wife is a retired physician whose practice for the last twenty years, before retiring, was in preventative medicine. I'm a retired lawyer and have been so for about three years. One day my wife was describing to me a method of lifting with which I was unfamiliar. She said that she had recently read a book titled *Body by Science* which recommended working out for a limited time—once a week and no more. She said that the authors of the book had significant success using high-intensity training methods and these were limited, on average, to once a week sessions. She suggested that I read the book. Now, over the years I've been regularly going to the gym three to six times a week. I'd usually be there for 1.5 to 3 hours. I was very curious to see what type of workout would safely bring gains doing it only once per week.

My mindset had difficulty wrapping around the once-a-week concept. Part of my problem was probably related to the fact that I'd spent over 50 years doing intense workouts—at least I thought they were intense. Counting the time going to and from the gym, changing clothes, the workout itself and showering, my workouts probably averaged 3 hours 5 times a week. That works out to 15 hours a week and does not include drive time to and from the gym. That translates to 780 hours (or 32.5 days) per year. Over 50 years that's 39,000 hours (or 1,625 days). Put another way that's 4.45 years-a fair chunk of my life! I do not consider these hours wasted, but from what I've learned, and since experienced, they might have been very inefficient.

My wife then told me that these high-intensity workouts could be completed in as little as 12-15 minutes per week. This was a bit more than I could stomach. After all, I had been lifting for many years and had a body of knowledge, based on research and actual experience, she did not possess. However, I also had tremendous respect for what my bride had to say on most any subject. She is typically well informed and well researched. After all, she was just asking me to read the darn thing. After *several months*, I did just that.

While I was reading the book I continued working out my normal 3 to 5 times a week. I should probably mention that

10

during the course of my weightlifting life I have experienced my share of weightlifting related injuries. Sprains, strains, joint problems and muscle tears dotted my weightlifting life. These injuries often caused me to modify my weightlifting routines while the associated parts of my body healed. I once tore the three triceps muscles in my right arm during a lifting workout. My orthopedist, who specialized in sports related injuries, said that he had never seen all three triceps muscles torn at one time. He said it was unlikely, due to the severity of the tears, that I would recover full use of the triceps. Fortunately, I did recover full use of all three triceps muscles, but the healing time was approximately 6 months. After that six-month period of time I had to begin anew strengthening muscles. Recovery time for associated sprains, strains and joint issues was typically much less. If however, I tried to come back from an injury too soon recovery time was always extended.

There were many benefits touted in the *Body by Science* book. Some of those benefits are the following:

1. Causes more muscle growth
2. Increases the storage reservoir for glucose in the muscles
3. Enhances insulin sensitivity which prevents or reverses diabetes
4. Helps reverse Metabolic Syndrome, a cluster of conditions:
   - Increased blood pressure
   - High blood sugar level, insulin resistance
   - Excess body fat around the waist
   - Abnormal cholesterol levels
   - This cluster of conditions increases the risk of heart disease, stroke and diabetes
5. Strengthens the heart
6. SuperSlow™ exercise stimulates growth of the fast-twitch muscle units, which in turn stimulates the release of growth hormone which in turn stimulates the growth of fast-twitch fibers. A good cycle!
7. Strengthens the Muscular Girdle
8. Stabilizes the Skeletal System

These are, undoubtedly, very important benefits, but the one that really caught my eye was the assertion that lifting, using the super slow method properly, would reduce the chance of strains, sprains and muscle injuries. Having experienced each of these conditions many times over the course of my exercise life this one really jumped out at me. I decided, "What the heck? I'll give it a try".

Since I retired I work out at home. Our equipment consists of a set of weights (power blocs) and a total gym (the machine advertised by Chuck Norris) supplemented by dumbbell plates. I structured my exercises to, as close as possible, target the same muscle groups as those recommended in the book. There were a couple of areas that I did not follow the recommendations in the book. I started off with very light weights to ensure that the range of motion I would be using was a comfortable range of motion for me and would not cause injury if done properly. I did, and still do, five basic exercises:

1. Seated row (on the total gym)
2. Chest press (with dumbbells)
3. Pull down (on the total gym)
4. Overhead press (with dumbbells)
5. Stiff-legged dead lift (with dumbbells). I have had a total knee replacement, or would have opted for squats.

It has now been almost three years since I started doing exercises using the super slow method. My workouts take from 13 to 18 minutes. I do 5 to 7 reps of each exercise. Each rep takes from 16 to 24 seconds. I typically do them about once every seven days. When I first started I was in reasonably good shape and found that a period of about 10 days elapsed before I felt I could do another workout. I have experienced increased strength and endurance. I do no other weightlifting, except chores on our property and hoisting a grandchild every now and then.

I had a concern that the exercises I was doing were not providing sufficient work to my abdominals and low back. My oldest daughter writes a blog and has regular Facebook postings for her health-related business. She recently posted a challenge, to those who read her business Facebook postings, regarding the planking exercise. The challenge was to, over a period of time, work up to a 3 minute plank. On the first day you were supposed to hold the plank as long as you could. I had performed the plank exercise many times over the years (usually as part of a lifting routine or cardio workout).

I know the plank to be an excellent core exercise and thought I'd give it a shot. Due to the fact that I had limited my exercises to the five previously mentioned (combined with my doubts as to their effect on core muscles) I did not expect to be able to hold the plank for long. Surprisingly, I held it for four minutes and could have gone longer. I now have no doubt that the five exercises I had been doing had a substantial effect on core muscle strength. My neck, chest, deltoids, arms, upper and lower back are all solid.

Body builders who try to build massive muscles and those folks, who take steroids and/or human growth hormones, seeking an increase in muscle mass, would probably not find this method of exercising attractive. Personally I have found the super slow method to be a healthy, safe, time efficient and productive way to exercise. *** End of Pat's story.

It Works for Us

So we embarked on our journey with SuperSlow™. Once I (Dr. Jo) finish my SuperSlow™ workout I feel good about having my muscle and heart conditioning done for the week. No more guilt about not exercising enough. And lots of time freed up to do other things.

But SuperSlow™ produces such a healthy strong body that I love to move it. In fact my muscles start feeling "stale" if I don't move them. It's like they're screaming, "Get up and move around. It's fun. It feels good". And so I do.

Now I can do something fun; dance, swim, bike, hike, jog, stretch, chase after my grandchildren or whatever. But keep in mind that this fun stuff does not push the muscles to the point of exhaustion because that would interfere with the rebuilding of the muscles that occurs after SuperSlow™.

In fact the SuperSlow™ gurus encourage folks to avoid any other exercise for the 5 to 7 days between SuperSlow™ workouts so the muscles have the opportunity to fully recover and increase to a greater strength level than they had prior to the last workout. On the other hand these experts also listened to and observed the folks they trained and realized that they've helped them create healthy fit bodies that can move and have a burning desire to move. So there's a healthy balance to be found between staying active without sabotaging muscle recovery after a SuperSlow™ workout. We will discuss this in more detail later.

After almost three years of SuperSlow™ strength training Pat and I are as fit as before and probably more fit with no injuries or joint, muscle, bone or ligament damage or inflammation. We have the strength to work hard physically around our mountain home developing and maintaining our garden, greenhouse and forest. Because of our rocky land we carry a lot of rocks, big and little, haul a lot of dirt, compost, straw and other garden material. In our seventies now, we may be stronger than we were in our forties.

In fact we just celebrated our 50th wedding anniversary. At our 25th wedding anniversary my wedding dress still fit and I wore it for a while during the celebration. I wondered, "Can I still fit into it at our 50Th anniversary?" I tried it on. Dang, I could fit it around my torso but my arms would not go into the snug fitting long sleeves as far as they needed to go.

But it wasn't because of fat! It's because I have muscles now that I did not have when I was younger, that I didn't have when I was 19 years old or 44 years old. I'm more fit now than I was then. I may be aging backwards. Let's age backwards together.

On average most Americans lose 1/2 pound of muscle per year and gain 1 pound of fat. Since the muscles burn 80% of calories losing muscle obviously sets you up to gain more fat if your intake of calories remains the same.

Progressively losing muscle also weakens you, makes you more prone to diabetes and bone fractures and less able to stay active and productive. So who's going to help you get off the toilet when your muscle strength deteriorates to the point you cannot even stand up without help?

But that's not you! You're eager to take responsibility for your own health and excited about the wonderful news that it only takes about 15 minutes a week to make such healthy gains in strength and improved metabolic functioning of your body. (SuperSlow™ workouts can take from 12 to 20 minutes in general.)

You may be thinking, "but I have never exercised before" or "I've never performed strength training exercises: can I actually do this?" The answer is a **Big Yes**. Remember that SuperSlow™ was created to be safe and do-able for elderly women with brittle bones and they increased their strength by 30% in 6 to 10 weeks, increasing more than the younger folks did who spent more time training but at a lesser intensity.

You've already realized that you cannot use the excuse "But I don't have time". Obviously that's a bunch of crock since it's only 12-20 minutes in a week on average.

That 12 to 20 minutes a week will bring you such great rewards in improving your health that you could actually gain time. How about less time at the doctor's office or in the hospital because of the improvement in your metabolism and the consequent decrease in obesity and the propensity for degeneration into disabling and killer diseases, especially the big 3, heart and blood vessel disease, diabetes and cancer.

How about feeling better mentally and physically, staying strong, active, and energetic and being filled with joy? How about investing 15 minutes per week in yourself and seeing the dividends grow? It doesn't get much better than that.

See if you can think of any 15 minute block of time in your daily routine that would garner you that much reward.

Is it worth it to you?

It Works

It works for us and it can work for you. We're passionate about sharing health and healthy living. We've seen folks build strong (not bulky) muscles and improve their health status by leaps and bounds. We know that engaging in SuperSlow™ can help people prevent or reverse the major killing diseases like heart disease, diabetes and cancer. That's exciting to us. We hope it's exciting enough to you that you will get started.

You invest only 15 minutes a week in yourself but that 15 minutes gives you such amazing benefits.

Let's proceed to learn the basics of performing the exercises and then find out more about the benefits to our physiology.

Just a word about terminology:

This muscle strengthening program has gone by many names over the years. So we weren't sure which names to use in this book. These are some of the names:

- super slow
- super-slow
- 10-10
- Slo-Mo™
- Ten/Ten™
- SuperSlow™

Also, various trainers and gyms have modified the program and given it other names. To keep his training method pure Ken Hutchins has the trademark for these three names: SuperSlow™, Slo-Mo™, Ten/Ten™.

In this book we follow the training methods as taught by Ken Hutchins and Dr. McGuff as closely as possible. To keep from infringing on the trademark of SuperSlow™ we will use the term super-slow or super slow when it's used in the research papers that we reference.

Also we will call this method Fit-in-15 in reference to our interpretation and implementation of this slow method of weight lifting for increased muscular mass and strength and all of the other benefits. Essentially SuperSlow™ and Fit-in-15 mean the same thing except Fit-in-15 emphasizes using free weights (dumbbells) and SuperSlow™ trainers may emphasize using weight machines, especially the Nautilaus machines.

If you want to view the SuperSlow™ method of training on machines go to Dr. McGuff's demonstration: http://www.youtube.com/watch?v=USyj-RgHFl0

http://www.youtube.com/watch?v=_tI4bOiSAaQ

Link to view other informative videos by Dr. McGuff:

http://www.bodybyscience.net/home.html/?page_id=2

CHAPTER 3
HOW TO PERFORM FIT-IN-15

Get ready—go for it. Time to learn the basics of the FIT-IN-15 exercise program.

Setting the Environment for Fit-in-15

Temperature

More good news! You don't have to sweat! Dr. McGuff says that sweating interferes with the process of completely fatiguing the muscles which you now know is so important to stimulate regeneration of more muscle.

So perform your Fit-in-15 workouts in a room that's around 63 degrees Fahrenheit (17 degrees Celsius). Now that's cool! Find a cool room with a good flow of cool dry air to prevent overheating.

A long time ago I didn't like to exercise because I didn't like to sweat. Water skiing suited me fine. When I got too warm I just let go of the ski rope and fell into that nice cool water. (Now I know that sweating is actually good for us because it helps detox those poisons. So I sweat while gardening or in the infrared sauna, but not during Fit-in-15!)

Clothing

Since you don't sweat during Fit-in-15 workouts, you can slip over to the gym for a workout during a break from work without taking the time to change clothes. Now that's another great benefit of Fit-in-15, so time efficient. You don't need a gym membership for Fit-in-15. This book is all about performing your workouts at home, keeping it time efficient and inexpensive.

Simply wear comfortable and flexible clothing to be able to perform the exercises correctly.

Free from Distractions

Fit-in-15 exercises require intense concentration so your workout room needs to be free of distractions such as:

- Music
- Mirrors
- Cell phones
- Pagers
- People that require attention
- Children that require attention

This time is just **for you.** Give yourself the luxury of that special just-for-you time. After all it's only 15 minutes per week. All that other stuff and those folks who depend on you can be taken care of after your special 15 minutes per week. By committing this time for yourself, you will be stronger and better able to minister to others as you become healthier. Your Fit-in-15 time is not a social event. Exercising together can be encouraging and can be part of your social life, but not part of Fit-in-15. It's a time to concentrate fully on each exercise and each rep! Have fun with other exercises as part of socializing.

Safety

For safety in lifting another person can spot for you. That person can be there to keep hands under the weights (without touching them) while you are lifting so they can grab them if your muscles fatigue to the point that you cannot lower them safely without hurting yourself. A spotter tends to be more important when using free weights. That person can be your encourager too, pushing you to maximally fatigue your muscles. A spotter can also assist you in performing the final rep or two.

The slow speed of movement of the weight, using correct form, protects the joints and muscles from injury.

A cool room prevents overheating.

Maintain proper alignment of head and neck to prevent headache and neck strain.

Breathe correctly.

Breathing Correctly is Essential to a Safe Workout

Folks have a natural tendency to hold their breaths when lifting weights, partly from concentrating on the intense lifting and partly to give them more power. But breath holding is dangerous. It creates increased pressure in the blood vessels. You know the dangers of high blood pressure for the heart and blood vessels. You don't want to blow a blood vessel in your brain, that's called a stroke, or in your heart or anywhere else.

Also the increased pressure in the blood vessels decreases the amount of blood returned to the heart. With less blood in the heart, there's less blood that the heart can pump out to the muscles. With blood deprivation your muscles cannot reach that desired state of complete fatigue. In other words, breath holding undermines your goal of completely fatiguing the muscles so that they can rebound to a higher level of mass and strength.

So, let's concentrate on proper breathing to prevent high blood pressure and to facilitate an optimal workout result.

How to breathe correctly:

- Breathe with your mouth open
- In a natural and continuous rhythm
- Breathe faster as you feel the burn in the muscle toward the end of each exercise

Stay Well-Hydrated

Drink plenty of water so the blood contains plenty of fluid to deliver nutrients to your cells and cart waste products away from the cells. Your muscles will recover and perform better when you are adequately hydrated.

Sleep

During sleep the muscles rest, relax, recuperate and rebuild. So get plenty of good sleep so these "4 Rs" can be effective in strengthening your muscles. Most folks require 7 to 9 hours of sleep each night to allow time for the body to regenerate and get rid of waste products.

We give you permission to sleep! In our culture we tend to glorify not sleeping to accomplish all these tasks that we think we have to finish. But in some ways that makes us slaves to "things". So relax, sleep well and awaken refreshed without feeling guilty!

Exercise is a Necessity

This intense exercise builds our bodies so we can enjoy the other activities of daily living.

"Exercise is not a luxury. It is a basic requirement for a normal healthy life." From Ken Hutchins PDF What is SuperSlow™.

Next review the following summary of the exercise set, so you see the simplicity of the program, then proceed to the details. Be sure to read the details before ever trying to perform the exercises so you understand the correct lifting methods and so you make the preliminary determinations before actually lifting the weights.

Overview of the Fit-in-15 workout:

Your exercise set only needs to include 4 to 5 exercises that utilize compound movements (activate many muscles at the same time). Now that's a compact workout.

Lift the weight through the range of motion taking 7-10 seconds, then return the weight to the starting point taking 7-10 seconds.

Perform each repetition 4-8 times until you absolutely cannot continue, then hold that resistance another 10 seconds. For greatest gain you need to **completely fatigue** your muscles. That means you absolutely cannot move that weight another fraction of an inch. Even if the weight is not moving when you reach that complete muscle fatigue, hold the resistance another 10 seconds if you possibly can.

Move quickly to the next exercise and repeat the process above until you have completed the 4 to 5 different exercises.

If you complete 5 different exercises in 12 to 15 minutes you will spend 2.5 to 3 minutes on each exercise including the time it takes to switch to the next exercise.

Before You Start

Another reminder: Always check with your doctor before starting an exercise program, especially if you are over 40 and have not been exercising regularly. You may want to share some of this written information with your doctor, especially in regards to the metabolic and strength enhancing benefits of this method of exercise, so he/she has a better understanding of the process, the safety of this exercise, and the health enhancing benefits for you.

Also review the American College of Sports Medicine recommendations before starting an exercise program on page 90 of this book.

The SuperSlow™ method can be utilized to aid recovery after an injury but definitely only under professional supervision by a doctor/physical therapist/chiropractor or other health professional because the program will need to be modified to accommodate the injury.

If You Have Never Lifted Weights

If you have not been trained in how to properly lift weights, find a personal trainer or someone with expert knowledge in weight lifting to help you learn the proper range of motion for each weight exercise you plan to use. Lifting without strict adherence to the correct method can cause injury. Injury of course can be very discouraging and might tempt you to quit, losing out on all of the wonderful health optimizing benefits. Only when you are very sure you can follow the correct protocol then you can continue your program without the supervision of a personal trainer or very knowledgeable weight lifter.

Have your trainer write down the proper positioning of your arms, hands, legs, feet, et cetera and the exact range of motion so you can refer to it when you're ready to begin your session. Go through each range of motion **without** holding any weights before you begin so the correct form is imprinted in your mind. Further on in this book you will find these written instructions for the exercises demonstrated in this book. Some people like to copy the information onto 3 x 5 cards to keep in their training area so they can review the proper form before each session.

You may want to work out with a buddy so you can encourage one another to press into that exercise just another few seconds to obtain maximum gain in strength. You can also spot for one another which can make the exercise even safer.

For Those Who Have Previously Engaged in Weight Lifting

If you have already enjoyed weight lifting prior to starting the Fit-in-15 program, it's still wise to make sure you use proper form. It's easy to get sloppy (at least for me). Here's what one experienced-at-weight-lifting doctor observed: "If you are an old pro at lifting then before each exercise run over in your mind what perfect form means. I like to take 5 seconds to read a card I have prepared that forces me to think about the few things that define" perfect form.

On the next few pages we will review the types of exercise equipment.

You don't have to run out and buy expensive equipment or belong to a gym for the Fit-in-15 workouts. Just keep it simple. Some people start by using cans of food. That may work with smaller cans, but dumbbell weights are a lot easier to grip.

You may be able to find sports stores that sell used dumbbells or start with a new set of smaller weights that increase from 1 pound up to 8 or 10 pounds. As you get stronger you can buy the next heavier weights that you need, spreading the cost over a greater time period.

Also consider visiting a gym or a friend that has a greater variety of sizes of dumbbells. Experiment with them to determine the weights you need before you buy yours so you don't waste your money on weights that are too light or too heavy for you. In the following pages you will learn how to determine your starting weight for each exercise.

Free Weights versus Machines

Intense strength training requires utilization of some kind of equipment in order to maximally stress your muscles. The possibilities include free weights, machine weights, or resistance bands.

Examples of Weight Strengthening Machines:

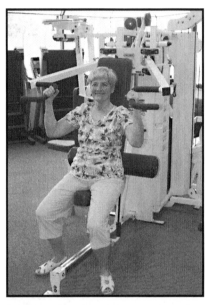

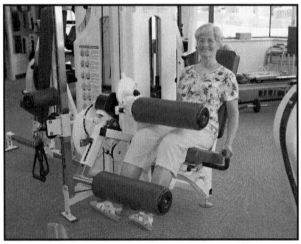

Examples of Free Weights

Dumbbells

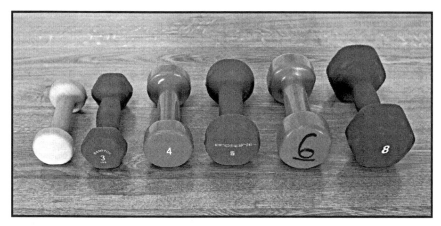

    These represent smaller sized dumbbells ranging from 2 pounds to eight pounds. As you get stronger you will gradually need to buy larger weights.

Barbells

The pictured barbell contains curves, another type of barbell has a straight bar.

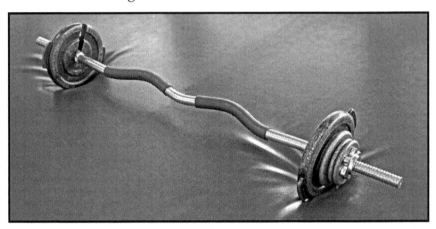

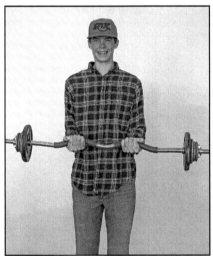 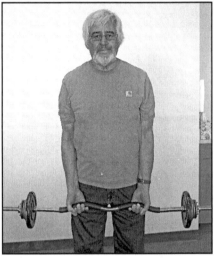

Trainers and lifters tend to have differences of opinion when it comes to choosing machines or free weights for SuperSlow™ training. Since SuperSlow™ exercises were originally developed for training folks on the Nautilus machines, many SuperSlow™ trainers and advocates highly recommend training on these machines.

Nautilus machines utilize cams to maintain tension on the muscles through the full range of motion. Machines made by other companies may or may not do so. Dr. McGuff prefers the use of the Nautilus machines because of this effect.

Don't start worrying about trying to find a gym with Nautilus machines. Other machines work well too and using free weights has a lot of advantages and may be the best choice. Obviously free weights cost a lot less to own than the machines. Unless you have a lot of money and space in your home, you're probably going to need to find a gym for your workouts if you want to use machines. Buying free weights is a lot less expensive than buying machines or joining a gym and you can work out in your own home. That alone saves time in getting ready and travelling to a gym.

There's a difference in movement between the two options as well. Your joints and limbs in normal activity move through three dimensions forward-backward, horizontally and vertically. So using free weights your joints and limbs can still move three-dimensionally giving you more functionality in daily living activities. Because of the potential to move in three dimensions you recruit more muscles fibers to stabilize free weights during the exercise. That means the smaller muscles that stabilize the larger muscles (like the gluteus and the hamstrings) strengthen along with the larger muscles keeping balance in your movements as you go about your daily routines of living. You're less likely to turn your foot and sprain your ankle when you step off a curb when these smaller stabilizing muscles strengthen along with the larger muscles.

When using machines you can only move in two directions so you don't recruit the smaller stabilizing muscles which can lead to an imbalance in your musculature. You may be more prone to twist your foot and sprain your ankle when stepping off a curb when your big strong gluteus, hamstring and calf muscles develop disproportionately to their stabilizing muscles. On the other hand if you want to develop your pectoral muscles so they stand out, machines would be your best choice to isolate that particular muscle during a workout. Also, if your muscles for some reason are out of balance, maybe after an injury on one side of your body, then a weight machine can isolate and specifically train the weaker muscle.

Because machines set the track for your movement you don't have to concentrate on the mechanics of the movement (form) and can concentrate more on moving slowly and intensely (the effort) through the exercise. Free weights require intense focus on form and thus may demand more concentration while exercising. Also machines may be safer to use, especially when exercising alone, because you have to have more control of a free weight to keep it from jerking you out of form and causing injury when you use a weight that is too heavy for you or if you become too fatigued to control it. However as you become stronger and competent in exercising with free weights the potential for injury lessens significantly especially when you always concentrate on optimal form of movement through the exercise.

Originally I thought that training on machines produced the best results in strengthening my muscles but now I feel that training with free weights produces the most balanced muscular results. That balance means I'm less likely to be injured when walking, lifting, cleaning, gardening and going about all my daily activities. So I don't have to join a gym. I can exercise at home. That's very convenient and easy on the budget and saves me a lot of driving time.

Working Out with Free Weights

Read completely through this explanation of how to perform the Fit-in-15 workout to get the overall picture. Then continue to read through and study the pictures providing the details of how to properly perform each weight exercise in the next section of this chapter. Only then will you be educated enough to safely start the Fit-in-15 program.

Step 1. Choose the 4 or 5 exercises for your workout. Since we want to develop balanced musculature we will choose exercises that engage one or more joints and activate the stabilizing muscles along with the larger muscles (compound movements). These are the exercises that we recommend and will demonstrate in the following pages:

- Bent-over dumbbell row
- Standing overhead press
- Stiff-legged dead-lift
- Bench press
- Squat

Step 2. Practice going through the proper form as you do each exercise before you ever add the free weights. When you can visualize the perfect form in your mind and move through it perfectly by memory, then add the weights.

Step 3. Determine how much weight you can lift, 1 pound, 5 pounds, 10 pounds or more. For beginners work with your personal trainer or knowledgeable weight lifter to make this determination. The starting weight will probably be a lot less than you imagine. The slow movement of the weight requires a lot more effort than using momentum to jerk the weight up. That intense effort quickly tires the muscle. If you decide to find your starting weight on your own it will take some trial and error. Start with light weights. If you can slowly lift that weight more than 8 repetitions without total fatigue, then you need to increase the weight. If your muscle is totally fatigued after only 3 repetitions, then decrease the weight.

Step 4. After determining the correct starting weight, reduce it by 30% for your first few workouts. "Before you start a super-slow workout," Hutchins says, "it's important to determine how much weight you can lift and then reduce it by 30%. If you're a novice and we knew the weight that was perfect for your strength it wouldn't be good to go that high," he says. "You need to master the technique."[i] Another reminder that proper technique is the priority at this stage of your "remodeling". We're not in a race. We're in a process that takes time. A well designed start produces well designed results. Start low, go slow and build up to full intensity of effort and weight.

Step 5. **Correct weight**—When you have found the right weight and lifted 30% less for a couple of weeks go ahead and increase the weight to the full amount appropriate for you for each exercise.

Step 6. **Speed**—As a general rule moving the first inch should take about 2 seconds. Take an additional 7 to 10 seconds to complete the extension or contraction. Then take 7 to 10 seconds to reverse the movement. The slowness and smoothness of this lifting motion protects the joints from injury because you naturally use less force as you fatigue. With less force you're not as prone to rip or tear tissues.

Step 7. **Repetitions**—Perform 4 to 8 repetitions of the exercise until you cannot do any additional repetitions (this is called complete failure of the muscles). Do not pause between repetitions. If you can only complete 3 repetitions decrease the weight at your next workout. If you complete more than 8 repetitions increase the weight at your next workout. Performing more than 8 reps means your effort was not intense enough to completely fatigue the muscle.

Breathing—Breathe through your mouth during each exercise—**Do not hold your breath**.

Step 8. Move quickly to the next exercise set only taking time to change the weight (for example from 10 pound weights for the chest press to 5 pound weights for the overhead press).

Frequency of Fit-in-15 Workout

By pushing your muscles to complete fatigue you give the muscles and the rest of your body such an intense stimulus that they have to adapt to it. They have to change. Given adequate rest between workouts the muscles will increase in size and metabolism will improve.

The key then is "adequate rest between workouts". You must rest long enough to allow the muscles to reach the maximum rebuilding level following the first workout. At your second workout you push your muscles to complete fatigue again. Rest again until they reach the maximum rebuilding level which will be a stronger level than after the first workout recovery. This process gradually builds muscles to a higher and higher strength.

How do you know when the muscles are ready for another workout? Listen to your body. Do your muscles still feel tired? Then wait another day or two. Weight lifting beginners may be ready for another Fit-in-15 workout in four days. More experienced lifters generally need seven days between workouts for muscle recovery. That seems strange doesn't it? But it makes sense when you realize that beginners have less muscle mass so the recovery is quicker for them. As you become stronger you can push more muscle mass to the maximum fatigue level; the intensity of the workout is greater; so it takes longer for them to replenish. At some point you will most likely reach the point of working out once per week.

If you work out more it's actually counter-productive. Folks who have engaged in weight lifting for years may really have trouble wrapping their minds around working out once per week for only 15 minutes until they understand the physiology of pushing the muscles to their max. Engaging in Fit-in-15 more frequently becomes a stress on the body that's working so hard to repair and rebuild those muscle fibers. Stress stimulates the adrenals to release cortisol which breaks down muscle to provide the protein that the body uses elsewhere to deal with the stress.

Therefore, working out again before your muscles have reached their full recovery defeats your whole purpose in gaining muscle mass and strength. Over training interferes with the adaptation response. And you waste your time. Your success comes from working with the physiology of your body to achieve your goals and allowing the adaptation response adequate time to complete the repair and rebuilding cycle.

This doctor explains it this way:

"I have also come to believe based on my experience over the past 2 years you won't see results quickly if you over train. In other words you need the time for the biochemistry to work and to let the damage you are producing heal. If you sprain an ankle (a big injury, not a micro injury) it doesn't get better in 2 days it gets better in 3 to 6 weeks. In other words you need to give your body the real time it takes to heal and that is based on its own physiology, not on some artificial schedule of lifts per week." From MD Amazon Review of *Body by Science*

Dr. McGuff tells us to not be religious about the time between intervals. I love his rule of thumb about determining the frequency of your workout: "So don't repeat the exercises on a set schedule. When it's time, you should feel like you're busting at the seams. You should feel so good that you feel you could turn a car over."

Some SuperSlow™ trainers actually told their clients to avoid doing any other type of exercise during the recovery phase. If they by chance saw a client out running, they would stop them and tell them to walk slowly back home. But then they began to realize that they were developing bodies like "Ferraris and telling them to drive in a 25 mph school zone". So there's a balance. You will find your balance as you work with the program.

Pat and I care for about 46 acres in the forest, a garden, a greenhouse, about 2,000 small evergreen trees that we had planted to reforest the land, cut our own wood, rake and move a lot of leaves, and haul rocks amid other measures of taking care of property. Sometimes we're involved in some heavy physical labor. At those times we do not engage in a Fit-in-15 workout. Our muscles need time to recover from those activities first.

You will learn to listen to your body and pace yourself appropriately too.

Most of the time though my body wants to move! My muscles feel stale and my blood sluggish if I sit too much (which by the way is not healthy for us and my body tells me about it). So I really enjoy swimming or biking or even jogging a couple of times per week.

If you want to "move it" too, then do something you enjoy. There's lots to do in the great outdoors and the sun and fresh air are so good for you. Have a great time. However, it's better to wait 2 days after Fit-in-15 before doing something fun and to rest at least one day before your next Fit-in-15.

Dumbbell Exercises

Now it's time to put what you've learned into action.

Remember to go through the range of motion for each dumbbell exercise without holding any dumbbells at first until you achieve the perfect form throughout the range of motion as described below. Since a picture is worth a thousand words look at the form of each person in the pictures as you practice the range of motion.

When you master the form, then hold some light weights and practice the form again. Gradually add more weight until you reach the amount of weight that completely exhausts your muscles in 4 to 8 repetitions of the lifting motion. For the first couple of weeks lift 30% less weight. When your muscles feel stronger increase to the level that totally exhausts the muscles in 4 to 8 repetitions.

SUPER SLOW DUMBBELL EXERCISE SET

Please pay special attention to the position of your palms during these exercises. In most of the exercises your palms should be facing one another. The chest press is the exception in this first set of five exercises. Your palms face your knees when performing the chest press.

Also notice the arm position for the Over Head Press. Keep them in front of your shoulders, palms facing one another. This position protects the rotator cuff. Many folks perform the Over Head Press with their arms wide apart and palms facing forward, a position that may cause injury to the rotator cuff.

If you start to use any of the additional exercises, study the position of your palms in each exercise as their position varies or changes in these exercises.

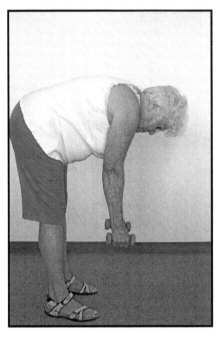

Bent-Over Dumbbell Row

Take hold of each dumbbell at shoulder-width apart with palms facing each other.

Bend over at the waist (keep your back straight) until your upper body is perpendicular to your lower body. Keep a slight bend in your knees to prevent straining your lower back.

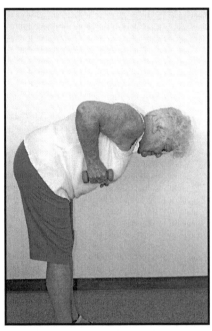

Slowly draw your arms upward until the dumbbells are just below neck level. Pause briefly in this fully contracted position, and then lower the dumbbells slowly back to the starting position. Repeat until failure of muscles.

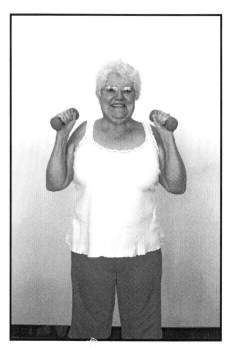

Standing Overhead Press

Can be performed standing or seated.

Take hold of each dumbbell with a shoulder width grip, and pull them up until you are holding them with your palms facing each other at the front of your shoulders.

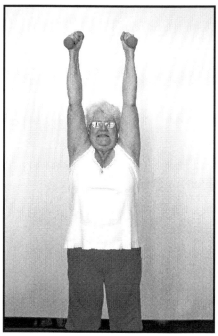

Keeping your back straight, slowly press the dumbbells overhead. Unlike the bent-over row, do not pause at the position of full contraction with this exercise, as your arms would be fully locked out, allowing the load to come off the muscles and onto the bone-on-bone tower. Slowly lower the dumbbell down to your shoulders. Repeat until failure.

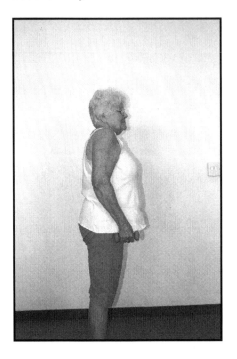

Stiff-Legged Dead Lift

Stand erect, with your feet about 16" apart.

Hold dumbbells at your side with your palms facing each other.

Keep your back straight, head up, hips and knees locked.

Bend forward until dumbbells touch floor (or as far as you can).

Return to starting position.

Repeat until failure of muscles.

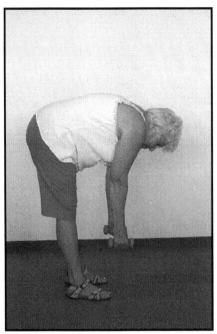

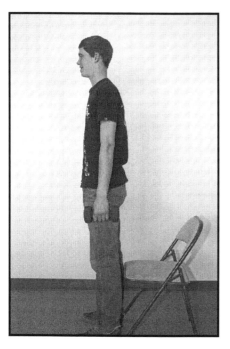

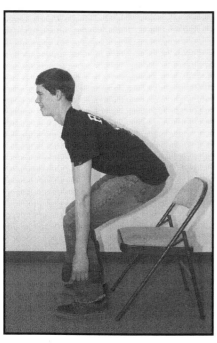

Squat

With a chair behind you, stand with your heels at the end of the chair.

Hold the dumbbells at your sides, at arm's length, palms facing each other. Keep your head up, back straight, feet firmly on the floor about 16" apart.

Squat until your buttocks touch the chair seat.

IMPORTANT—Keep your knees behind your toes. Do not sit on the chair, keep tension on the thighs. Keep your knees close together. Return to the starting position. Repeat until failure of muscles.

Pat and Dr. Jo Tillman

Chest Press

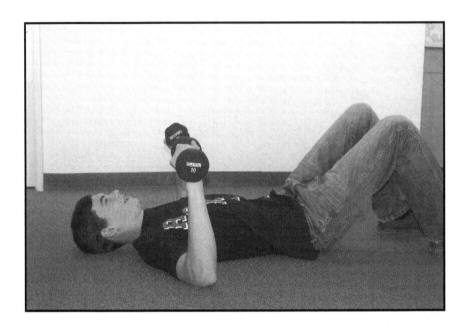

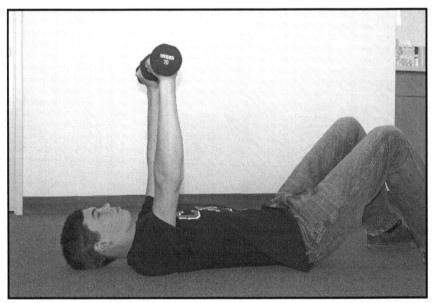

Chest Press Instructions

Can be performed on a bench or the floor

Laying on your back, hold a dumbbell in each hand in line with your chest, about shoulder width apart and with palms facing out toward your feet.

Press the dumbbells up above your chest until your arms are locked out.

Do not pause in this position; if you do, as would happen with the overhead press, the load will be transferred onto the bone-on-bone tower that results from locking out your arms, rather than being placed on the musculature responsible for moving your arms into this position.

Slowly lower the dumbbells until they reach the position you started from.

Repeat until failure of muscles.

ADDITIONAL FIT-IN-15 DUMBBELL EXERCISES

Periodically your mind and your muscles need a change to keep you interested and to improve the performance of your muscles. Substitute one or more of the following exercises into your workout.

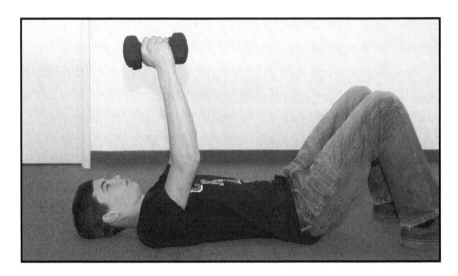

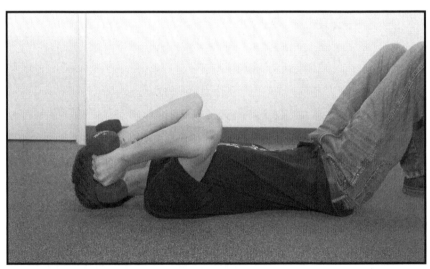

Lying 2 Arm Triceps Dumbbell Curl Instructions
Works triceps muscles on back of upper arms

Lie on back on bench or on the floor.

Hold dumbbells at arms' length above your shoulders.

Lower dumbbells in semicircular motion, bending arms at elbows, keeping upper arms vertical until dumbbells are parallel to ears.

Return to starting position.

Repeat until failure of muscles.

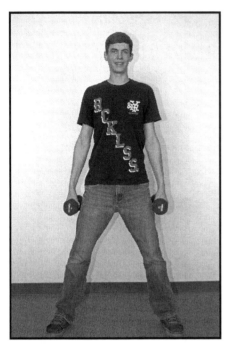

Cross-Over 2 Arm Dumbbell Touches

Works Oblique & Lower Back Muscles

Replaces Stiff-legged Dead Lift in your routine

Stand with legs about 30 inches apart

Hold dumbbells in each hand.

Bending at waist touch left hand dumbbell to right foot (or as close as you can get), and return to upright position.

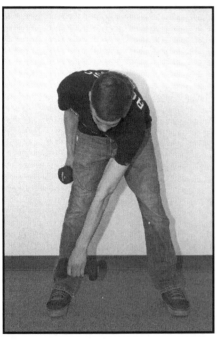

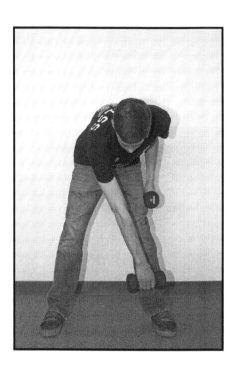

**Cross-Over 2 Arm
Dumbbell Touches**
Continued

Repeat with right hand dumbbell.

Repeat right and left touches to failure of muscles.

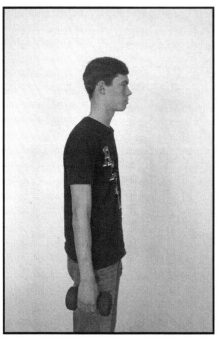

Standing 2 Arm Dumbbell Curls

Works Biceps & Arms

Stand erect with feet about 16" apart.

Keep your back straight, eyes front, hips and legs locked.

Start with dumbbells at arms' length, palms in, at sides of upper thighs.

Begin curl with palms in until past upper thighs, then turn palms up for remainder of curl to shoulder height.

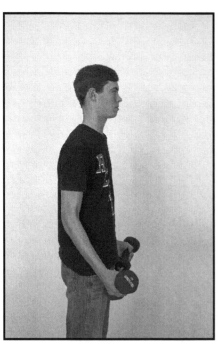

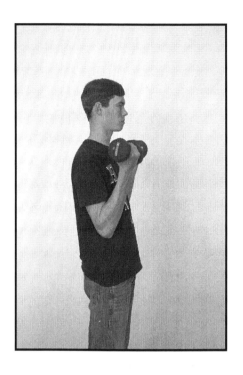

Standing 2 Arm Dumb-bell Curls
Continued

Keep upper arms close to sides while lifting dumbbells up to shoulder level.

Keep palms up while lowering past thighs then turn palms in and finish in start position.

Repeat to failure of muscles.

If you would like to keep records of your progress Pat created some wonderful forms that you can download. One master form has the first five exercises printed on it and the other is left blank so you can write in whatever exercises you are engaged in. An explanation of how to interpret and use the forms accompanies them in the download which you can find here:

http://www.drjomd.com/products/fit-in-fifteen-workout-logs/

The Plank

Since Pat mentioned The Plank exercise in his "**ONE MAN'S EXPERIENCE WITH SUPERSLOW™ WEIGHT TRAINING—by P.J. Tillman**" on page 10 and since it's such a great exercise for the core (central) muscles of the body, we're going to introduce it to you. Perhaps you will want to utilize it in your workout at some point.

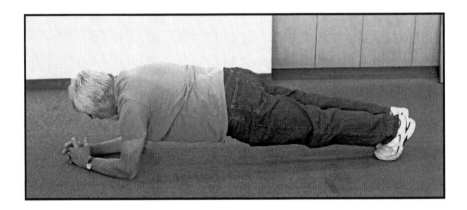

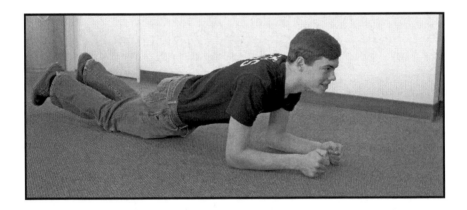

The Plank Instructions

We believe that a properly done plank is one of the best exercises for the development of core muscles. The standard plank, which is pictured on the previous page, primarily engages the abdominals and the back muscles which run from the head to the lower back. Also engaged, but to a somewhat more limited extent, are the trapezius and rhomboid muscles in the back; shoulder rotator cuffs and deltoids and the chest pectorals. The quads in your legs and your gluteus (butt muscles) also receive some serious work. Assuming proper form, the amount of development of the involved muscles is dependent on how long you are able to stay in the plank position and, to a somewhat lesser extent, how often you perform this exercise.

How to do a Standard Plank

1. Start lying face down on the floor
2. Rest your upper body on your elbows with your forearms pointing forward and your hands palms down flat on the floor. Your upper arm should be straight down from your shoulders and your upper arm should be at a 90 degree angle to your lower arm (as pictured).
3. Keeping your body in a straight line rise onto your toes. Keep your upper arms straight down from your shoulders and take care not to raise or lower your butt. Keep your back completely straight and tighten your abdominals.
4. Maintain that position for as long as you are able. Start by holding the plank position for 15 seconds. At your next time interval for the plank increase to 30 seconds. Continue to increase the time spent in the correct, body-in-a-straight-line-position as you are able to. You may recall that Pat held the plank position for four minutes when he tested the strength of his core muscles after participating in the Fit-in-15 muscle strengthening program for several months. Holding a plank for 4 minutes is a long time and really hard to do. So, don't feel

disappointed if you can only hold it 15 to 30 seconds at first. You're a champ for starting the process of building up your core muscles.

5. You can "cheat" and hold the position a lot longer if you lift your butt higher. I accidentally did that for a while and thought I was really doing well. When someone showed me that I was not holding my body in a straight line, I corrected it and found out it's a lot harder when done properly and a lot better for strengthening your core. So have someone take a look at your alignment to help you make sure you're keeping all parts tucked in with butt and abs engaged.

A standard plank may be too difficult for some folks. Not to worry, you can reduce the difficulty by performing a plank from your knees, as pictured. Notice that the feet are lifted off the floor when on your knees for this beginner's plank position. You can work up to a standard plank as your muscles get stronger. It can also be done with your arms fully extended in the push up position.

There are many other forms of the plank such as a side plank, a plank done while lifting one leg or one arm, etc. Start with the standard plank - it's a great exercise.

Those who plank together grow old together.

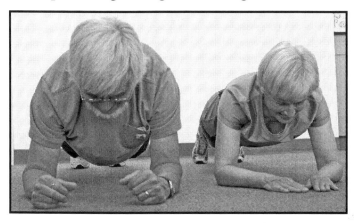

Now that you're excited about your Fit-in-15 workout program you may want to keep track of your progress using these workout logs.

Download them from this link. You have our permission to make copies of them for your personal use.

http://www.drjomd.com/products/fit-in-fifteen-workout-logs/

CHAPTER 4
THE OTHER AMAZING BENEFITS
OF THE SUPERSLOW™ WORKOUT

If the benefit of gaining and maintaining an optimal level of fitness in only 15 minutes per week isn't enough to get you dedicated to doing it, take a look at these other amazing benefits, ones you might never imagine were quietly going on in your metabolism as you strengthen your muscles. All of these benefits have been documented by high quality researchers like Ken Hutchins and Dr. Doug McGuff.

First of all let's understand how SuperSlow™ training builds muscles in contrast to how endurance training (prolonged exercise programs like running, biking or swimming a long time) affects them. Muscles contain 3 basic types of fibers named by how fast they fatigue. Slow twitch fibers take a long time to fatigue, intermediate twitch fibers take an intermediate time to fatigue and the fast twitch fibers fatigue the fastest.

Slow twitch fibers contain smaller units of muscle cells that use oxygen to convert glucose into energy. Therefore they activate during aerobic (using oxygen) types of activity and they recover quickly. When you exercise at the level of feeling a little short of breath but still able to talk, you maintain adequate oxygen delivery for the slow twitch fibers to continue to function. At that level with proper conditioning you can run a long time. You can "endure". So long distance running, biking, or cross-country skiing, etc. is called endurance exercise.

If you drive your muscles beyond the capacity of your heart, lungs and blood vessels' ability to deliver oxygen to these muscles they then switch to anaerobic (without oxygen metabolism). At this phase the intermediate fibers kick into action, with more effort in exercise the fast twitch fibers activate.

Fast twitch fibers utilize very little oxygen in converting glucose to energy so they take longer to recover. They can only function for short, intense periods of exercise. But that short intense time produces an abundance of health enhancing properties for your body since the fast twitch fibers:

1. Efficiently produce more muscle mass
2. Are the largest reservoir in your body for storing glucose
3. Cause your cells to be more sensitive to insulin helping to reverse diabetes and metabolic syndrome
4. Burn a lot more calories than the slow or intermediate twitch fibers

By stressing your muscles to the maximum effort with the SuperSlow™ workout you stimulate the growth of the fast twitch muscles, the power house of improving your metabolism and health. On the other hand, endurance type exercise causes the fast twitch fibers to atrophy. In the economy of the body the fast twitch fibers are expensive to maintain. They require a lot of calories. If you don't use them you lose them. The body lets them fade away unless the muscles receive that maximal stimulus of complete fatigue (failure) periodically.

Because endurance-type exercises do not stress the muscles enough to stimulate the growth of fast twitch fibers a big loss of body tissue occurs. Endurance participants lose muscle mass. Look at dedicated distance runners. They usually appear very lean and thin. The body adapts to the activity of the person. With less weight runners can run longer and farther but at what cost? They've lost a lot of muscle tissue. They've lost the fast twitch fibers, the high-quality fibers that hold the largest amount of glucose in the storage form known as glycogen. Couch potatoes beware. Not exercising at all causes a faster rate of decline in the glucose-insulin regulating processes of the body.

Loss of the glucose reservoir capacity leads to loss of insulin sensitivity at the cell membrane. Without fast twitch muscle fibers the body has decreased ability to store the glucose that enters the blood stream. The cells don't want to drown in glucose inside the cell, so their cell membranes resist the action of insulin, the hormone that attaches to the cell membrane to facilitate the entrance of glucose into the cell. Since high blood glucose signals danger to the endocrine system, the pancreas responds by squirting out more insulin. Gradually blood glucose (sugar) and insulin levels climb too high, a set up for the development of the Metabolic Syndrome.

Reversing or Avoiding Metabolic Syndrome
Syndrome refers to a cluster of conditions. So, metabolic syndrome refers to a cluster of conditions that precede the overt development of heart disease, Type 2 Diabetes, kidney disease or stroke. Reversing this syndrome before it becomes that pathological can prevent a lot of pain, disability and even death. Over 1/5th of the people in the USA have upset their body metabolism to the point of carrying around this ticking time bomb of deranged physiology. (On the bright side, the percentage of Americans with Metabolic Syndrome decreased from 25.5% in 1999 to 22.9% in 2010.)[7]
Here's that unhappy cluster of conditions:

- Increased blood pressure
- High blood sugar, insulin resistance
- Too much fat around the waist
- Abnormal cholesterol levels
- Abnormal blood triglyceride levels

Do you see yourself in this cluster of conditions? Many people go merrily about their daily living without realizing the jeopardy they have put themselves in. They often do not realize that they are carrying around this cluster of conditions known as the Metabolic Syndrome, in other words, messed up metabolism.
Would you be willing to invest 15 minutes of your time every week to reverse this condition and stave off those degenerative diseases, those big killers, heart disease, stroke and Type 2 Diabetes? Wouldn't it be worth it to you to spend that time in the SuperSlow™ weight strengthening exercises to reverse your insulin resistance, increase your glucose

storage capacity, decrease your waist line fat and stabilize your blood fats. Just kick Metabolic Syndrome out the door!

Remember that insulin resistance refers to the decreased ability of insulin to usher glucose across the cell membrane to the inside of the cell where it is burned in the mitochondria to produce energy. The cell decreases the size of the "door" into the cell. It says, "Enough is enough. I'm overwhelmed by all of this glucose (sugar). I can only turn so much of it into energy."

SuperSlow™ decreases insulin resistance at the cell membrane by stimulating the production of more fast twitch muscle fibers that love to turn glucose into glycogen, the storage form of carbohydrates (sugars) in the body and then burn that glycogen for energy when the body demands it. The greater the increase in fast twitch muscle fibers, the greater the glucose storage capacity. These new cells are receptive to the actions of insulin, are sensitive to insulin. So SuperSlow™ helps turn insulin resistance into insulin sensitivity. The sugar now has a healthy place to go instead of being shuttled into fat storage leading to excess fat around the waist.

Fast twitch muscle fibers also burn the most calories of any tissue in the body and they require those calories not only during the intense exercise of SuperSlow™ but also during the rest of the day and night. Utilizing glucose properly allows the fat around the waist (and all other parts of the body too) to slowly dissipate around the clock.

See how Metabolic Syndrome gradually disappears as you persist in improving your metabolism with SuperSlow™.[8]

Of course, eating "clean" has to be incorporated into your lifestyle habits too. We will talk about healthy eating later.

If you're in the other 80% of the population that does not have the conditions associated with Metabolic Syndrome, congratulations. Incorporating SuperSlow™ in your lifestyle habits will give you more insurance against ever developing it.

Increase Your Own Human Growth Hormone (HGH)

Our hormones tend to decrease as we age and that's true for Human Growth Hormone (HGH) too. We drop into

"Somatopause". When that happens the effects of HGH on our tissues decrease too. That's a bummer since HGH has these functions:

Stimulates increased production of proteins which can increase muscle mass

Helps break down body fat and maintain good lean to fat ratio in body[9]

Increases intestinal absorption of calcium, helping maintain strong bones[10]

Therefore some doctors administer injections of HGH for increasing muscle mass and decreasing body fat in their aging patients. This practice is controversial and quite expensive costing $400 to $500 per month. [11]

But you get this fabulous "side-effect" of increased HGH production from SuperSlow™ workouts. It increases your HGH levels without having to pay anything for it except 15 minutes of your time once per week. It's one of those wonderful bio-feedback cycles in your body. The fast twitch fibers must have growth hormone to produce more of them so they can produce a lot of power. In the feedback loop fast fibers promote the production of growth hormone. So, SuperSlow™ exercise stimulates growth of the fast-twitch muscle units, which in turn stimulates the release of growth hormone which in turn stimulates the growth of fast-twitch fibers. A good cycle![12]

Lose Fat Faster

SuperSlow™ exercise helps burn fat in several ways.

1. SuperSlow™ workouts stimulate increased production of your own Human Growth Hormone (HGH). More HGH mobilizes more fat.

2. SuperSlow™ workouts increase the number of fast twitch muscle fibers. These fibers require a lot of calories just to maintain them. So even at rest the body burns more calories when the fast twitch muscle mass increases. Actually the amount of calories burned during exercise (even the long boring kind) does not contribute as much to fat loss as the

continual burn of fat that occurs with increased muscle mass throughout the day and even while you're sleeping.[13]

Dr. Al Sears discusses fat burning in his PACE program (a type of High Intensity Interval Training that's a bit different than SuperSlow™). Long-duration exercise burns fat *during* your workout. **But** your body thinks, "Oh I need a reserve of fat available all the time so I have the fuel to burn the next time this dude exercises." So your body promises to store more fat every time you exercise. Then you have to burn it all up again with those long work-out sessions.

That's why Dr. Sears advocates for short workout sessions as little as 10-12 minutes and never over 20 minutes. In these short sessions the body does not have to click into burning fat. It simply burns the carbs (glucose, glycogen) out of the muscles which triggers the "after burn". Only after you stop the PACE short exercise session (also known as High Intensity Interval Training) does your body start to burn fat and continues to burn fat for 24 hours after your session. You continue to develop more muscle tissue that needs fuel continuously all day every day, muscles that burn 80% of calories when you eat appropriately for optimal health.

Dr. Al Sears says, "After a while, your body stops making fat all together-it simply doesn't need it anymore! This after burn is the key to getting rid of excess body fat—not long hours of boring exercise."

Dr. Doug McGuff gives us another explanation for how SuperSlow™ helps us lose fat faster. He thought morbidly obese people might have big muscles under the fat but, no, they have paper-thin muscles. Any stretching tears the muscle producing pain. If that muscle tear occurs in the kidney area doctors think of kidney problems. But actually that flank pain comes from the fragility and tearing of the muscle overlying the kidneys. To compound the problem these obese folks cannot build up the muscles because they have internal starvation from not having the capacity to store glucose as glycogen. Since they lack the fast twitch muscles that are the tanks for glucose, anything that they eat goes immediately to fat. And they are always feeling starved! Now that's a vicious cycle to break out of.

How do they turn this dilemma around? SuperSlow™ to the rescue again because it aggressively empties sugar out of the muscle cells. As the fast twitch fibers increase, they hold more glucose in the form of glycogen. This increased glucose storage capacity gives the glucose a place to go. It no longer has to be shuttled to fat storage. The fat accumulation stops and then begins to decrease. Combined with eating a low carbohydrate diet (more emphasis on protein and fat in meals) they bring their metabolism into a healthy state of functioning and can grow more muscle to burn up that fat. What a great way to lose fat faster!

Ken Hutchins sums up the fat loss this way. "Some people exercise because it burns a few calories," Hutchins said. "That's not a good reason to exercise. Replacing fat tissue for muscle tissue is what burns calories. Every pound of muscle tissue gained requires 50 more calories a day."

Thus, said Hutchins, "A woman who can replace 10 pounds of fat with 10 pounds of muscle not only will drop two dress sizes, she will burn 500 more calories per day, even on days she does not exercise."[14]

A current research study divided 45 women into 3 exercise groups. One group engaged in high-intensity intermittent exercise (HIIE). The second group performed "steady-state exercise" (exercise exertion remained the same throughout the session, so they had to remain in the aerobic (oxygen-using) form of activity). The third group did not exercise at all and so was the "control group". Both exercise groups significantly increased their cardiovascular fitness. But only the HIIE (high-intensity) group had significant reductions of their total body fat, especially on their legs and trunks and a decrease in their fasting plasma insulin levels.[15]

Looks to me like high intensity strength training provides an abundance of benefits compared to endurance type exercises. So why not **spend less time more intensely** to reap a host of benefits that you don't get with other types of exercise?

Builds Structural Integrity

Increasing the size of your muscles builds up your muscle mass, the total amount of muscle in your body. But never fear. You most likely won't develop big bulky muscles. Body builders spend hours and hours in the gym to build those bulky muscles and not everyone has the genetic makeup to build big muscles. Developing big bulky muscles is not our goal in this muscle strengthening program. Our goal is to have a healthy amount of muscle tissue and strength because maintaining muscle mass and strength provides so many benefits to keep us strong and healthy throughout our entire lives.

Building muscle may not actually increase the size of your arms or your thighs. For as you build muscles you tend to lose fat. Since muscle is more compact than fat the size of your arms or legs may actually decrease when you measure the circumference of your arm or leg. On the other hand if you have skinny little arms and legs and you build up the muscles you most likely will have larger arms and legs when you measure their circumference. And that's most likely a good thing. You will start to look healthy and trim and fit.

By increasing muscle size you actually build more body armor. This body armor acts like a girdle to stabilize your bones, ligaments, joints and spine. Folks who have healthy muscle strength but thin bones are far less likely to break a bone if they fall because of the protection of the muscles. Also good muscle strength and mass improves balance which decreases the propensity to fall.

Spending only 15 minutes of exertion per week provides insurance against the loss of muscle mass as we age. Researchers have found that skeletal muscle loss begins at age 20 and continues until the end of life. From age 20 to 80 years of age there's a 30% reduction in muscle mass due to a decline in both the size and number of muscle fibers. But exercising counteracts this muscle fiber loss.[16]

In conjunction with the loss of muscle fibers people gain fat on a yearly basis unless they're exercising. You can see the problem. Loss of muscle fiber gives you less of the tissue that burns fat and thus the chronic problem with constant weight gain from year-to-year. But now you know how to counteract this vicious cycle of muscle loss and weight gain. All you have to do is exert yourself to the maximum with 4 to 5 different exercises once a week. How easy is that?[17]

Besides strengthening the muscles, SuperSlow™ exercises strengthen the bones even reversing osteoporosis. Actually Ken Hutchins originally developed the SuperSlow™ program to help older women with frail bones increase their bone density. Indeed they significantly increased their bone density over just 6 to 10 weeks, a remarkable accomplishment.

Folks who have the same amount of bone loss can have a different propensity for breaking their bones because a strong muscle girdle protects and strengthens these frail bones. You've probably noticed people that have the so-called "dowager's hump" where their shoulders are slumped forward and they have a big hump on the upper part of their backs just below their necks. That occurs because they've lost strength in the shoulder and upper back muscles allowing the shoulders to slump forward. This abnormal slump forward places a curvature into the upper thoracic spine causing abnormal pressure on the forward (anterior) portion of the vertebral body. This anterior compression compacts the front portions of them forcing them into a wedge shape with the thinner portion in the front if you look at the spinal x-rays from the side view. This pressure on that front part of the vertebra can lead to fractures that cause a lot of pain. We tend to see this more in women and I have seen some older women who are very disabled and in chronic constant pain from the abnormalities they had developed in their spine because of the lack of muscles. Strengthening our muscles can prevent this miserable disease.[18]

As the joints regularly move smoothly through the weight exercises they become more mobile leading to better functioning of the joints in everyday living. As the joints become more stable they are more protected from injury. SuperSlow™ also reduces the symptoms of arthritis, perhaps by just getting the fluid moving in the joints. However in my experience exercise mobilizes toxins out of tissues. SuperSlow™ exercise could very well help mobilize the toxins out of the joints. When toxins are in the tissues they cause inflammation which causes pain and swelling. Therefore removing the toxins helps reverse the pathology and the symptoms.

So you retain muscle and bone strength even into old age and reduce the risk of falls and broken bones. On top of that strengthening your muscles reduces and helps prevent lower back pain.[19] As you strengthen your muscles you gain more stamina for the daily activities of life like climbing stairs, or pulling weeds or just walking to your car or the mailbox. And you can have more fun doing the things you love best like swimming, dancing, skiing or biking. What a joy to be able to play with your grandchildren and explore exciting places. Those 15 minutes of exercise every week provides a whole world of benefits in daily living and enjoyable activities.

SuperSlow™ builds structural integrity into your body by:

- Increasing muscle mass and strength, [20]
- Providing a protective armor for the bones, joints and spine
- Strengthening bones, even reversing osteoporosis
- Improving joint movement increasing mobility
- Increasing joint stability and protection
- Reducing symptoms of arthritis
- Improving balance and decreasing propensity to fall down
- Retaining strength in old age thereby reducing the risk of falls and broken bones
- Increasing stamina for fun activities and activities of daily living
- Reducing and preventing lower back pain

Strengthens heart and blood vessels

Most of us have been conditioned to believe that we need to exercise for a prolonged period of time to improve our heart and blood vessel fitness, to do "cardio" workouts also known as "aerobics". However Dr. McGuff's research puts new light on that thought process. He explains that your cardiovascular system (heart and blood vessels) respond to the mechanical work of your muscles. Your muscles need to return an increased volume of blood to the heart so it can pump out more blood with each beat. In other words you want the heart to squeeze out a greater volume of blood with each heartbeat.

The cardiac output is determined by how fast your heart is beating (the heart rate) multiplied by how much blood is squeezed out with each heartbeat (the stroke volume). So the stroke volume equals the amount of blood ejected out of the left ventricle with each heartbeat.

CARDIAC OUTPUT = HEART RATE X STROKE VOLUME

Let's take a quick look at how the blood is pumped out of the heart into the blood vessels and back to the heart. The left ventricle squeezes the blood into the large arteries. The arteries become progressively smaller as they branch out to the periphery of the body supplying the tissues with oxygen and nutrients from the blood. Eventually they turn into capillaries which then return the blood to the small veins which flow into the larger veins which empty into the right upper chamber of the heart, the right atrium. The right atrium squeezes the blood into the right ventricle, the lower right portion of the heart which then squeezes it into the left atrium, the left upper portion chamber of the heart. And finally the blood is returned to the left ventricle.

Now that you understand how the blood flows through the heart and blood vessels let's get back to stroke volume because it's critical in understanding the difference between aerobic exercise and anaerobic exercise effects on the cardiovascular system. The stroke volume is directly proportional to the amount of the blood that returns to the right side of the heart. With sprint type exercises the muscular contractions are fast, short and choppy. That equates to lower volumes of blood being returned to the right side of the heart. So the left ventricle consequently receives less blood and the stroke volume goes down. The left ventricle squeezes out a smaller volume of blood.

In contrast the sustained and intense muscular contractions of SuperSlow™ deliver large amounts of blood back to the right side of the heart and out into the left ventricle. This process increases the stroke volume, the amount of blood that can be squeezed out with each heartbeat, thus improving the cardiac output. SuperSlow™ strength training strengthens the heart and the blood vessels making them more efficient. In contrast endurance or aerobic training is not as effective in conditioning the heart to an optimal level of fitness.

Strength training can also recondition the heart after a heart attack. However this training should be performed initially under strict medical supervision.

Many of us, including me, have used our heart rate while exercising and at rest as an indicator of our level of cardiac fitness and as a guide to how much to push ourselves during training. However cardiac output (a measure of cardiac fitness) involves 2 factors, both heart rate and stroke volume. We cannot measure our own stroke volume while working out. But stroke volume is the more important factor in evaluating cardiac fitness because cardiac output can be increased more by the stroke volume than the heart rate. So using the heart rate as a good indicator of cardiac fitness is not particularly helpful in determining your cardiovascular fitness according to Dr. McGuff. As a matter fact they don't even pay attention to heart rate in his gyms.[21]

If your heart's working better, you'll want your arteries to function better too. It takes both to pump the blood around the body and deliver oxygen to your tissues. Sure enough, high intensity exercise "enhances endothelial function" too. It improves the lining of your arteries and therefore decreases the chances of developing hardening of the arteries.[22]

Helps lower blood pressure

In the long term strengthening your muscles with weight training helps lower blood pressure. However during the actual act of lifting the weight your blood pressure may temporarily go higher. As a precaution always check with your doctor before you start a weightlifting program or any exercise program if you have high blood pressure.

The Mayo Clinic website cautions against weightlifting if your blood pressure is out-of-control, if it's higher than 180/100 mm Hg. Of course with a blood pressure that high you'll get to your doctor right away.

If your blood pressure is higher than 160/100 mmHg then ask your doctor what precautions you should take when weightlifting.

Blood pressure can spike dangerously high if you hold your breath while weightlifting. Therefore be sure to breathe easily through your mouth while going through the weightlifting maneuver. Be very conscious of your breathing during weightlifting because folks commonly hold their breath due to their intense concentration on lifting the weight properly. Focus on breathing in and out through your mouth during the contraction and exertion phase of the lift. Besides keeping your blood pressure under control proper breathing technique delivers optimal amounts of oxygen to your muscles.[23]

If you have high blood pressure, with your doctor's permission, persevere in your SuperSlow™ regimen and see what happens to your blood pressure. Most folks see a beneficial decrease to healthier levels.

Lowers your cholesterol LDL/HDL ratio and increases your HDL cholesterol

Despite an insane workout regimen Dr. Philip Alexander, MD could not get his HDL cholesterol above 42. HDL is the good guy in the cholesterol story. HDL of course stands for high density lipoprotein. You want your "Highs" high and your "Lows" low. As an internist this doctor knew that higher HDL levels indicate healthy benefits to the body.

He also knew that exercise helped increase HDL levels. So for 20 years he ran an average of 60 miles a week. On top of that he would bike another 35 miles. Even this good doctor knew he was nuts. Especially when he ran 50 full rounds up and down the football stands. To quote him, "Every joint hurt. The next day I felt like I had been run over by a truck."

Despite beating himself up this way his good HDL cholesterol was not increasing

"I didn't know how to get a more cardiovascular workout," he says, "I knew what I was doing wasn't working and it was tearing my body apart."

Then he discovered SuperSlow™ weight lifting and contacted Ken Hutchins. With guidance from Hutchins he learned how to exercise sanely. Now he gets all the cardiovascular and strength training he wants with a couple of SuperSlow™ sessions each week. And guess what? His HDL increased up to 62. Now he's exercising in a way that is kind to his body and gives him the benefits he was looking for.

His story is a great one to highlight the fact that SuperSlow™ exercise increases good cholesterol, HDL, and decreases the LDL/HDL ratio, all good benefits for healthy living.[24]

Decrease oxidative stress and increase anti-oxidant production

When Dr. Philip Alexander over exercised before he found SuperSlow™ he created high levels of oxidants, free radicals, that damaged his body. That's why he felt like he had been run over by a truck after those over training exercises.

But happily he found SuperSlow™ and now when he exercises wisely he no longer creates that oxidative stress on his body. In fact weight training can increase antioxidant production in the body that helps nullify free radicals that we daily encounter in our environment.

The next study was done with a slightly different type of high intensity training regimen, known as high-intensity interval training (HIIT). Eight fellows who were very active entered into a cycling training program. They peddled as hard as they could for 30 seconds then rested for four minutes. They repeated this cycle of 30 second high intensity peddling followed by 4 minutes of slower peddling 4 to 6 times during each HIIT session. After only three weeks of training their blood levels of antioxidants increased significantly and their blood markers of oxidative stress decreased significantly. Amazingly enough this all occurred after only nine training sessions and only 22 minutes of high-intensity exercise. The authors of this study concluded that short term HIIT has a positive "effect not only on physical conditioning but also on health promotion".[25]

Increases lung volume

High intensity training increases lung volume whereas lower intensity exercise does not. In one study folks exercised at 3 different intensity levels, 80% or 60% or 40% of maximum intensity and the fourth group did not exercise at all (the control group) for 8 weeks. The group exercising at 80% of maximum were the only ones who increased their lung volume.[26]

Another similar study demonstrated that high intensity exercise increases the thickness of the diaphragm (the large muscle that helps your lungs expand and contract with each breath), increased lung volume and exercise capacity in healthy people.[27] And another concluded that high intensity training increased respiratory muscular strength more effectively than endurance training with the added bonus of accomplishing greater respiratory strength in a shorter amount of time.[28]

Boost immunity and the ability to fight disease

In my research I ran across this concept, a nice surprise to me and an added bonus of strength training, in this quotation:

> "Given that muscles are major reservoirs for the body's supply of fuel in the form of amino acids, having more muscle also may mean having more fuel," said C. Jessie Jones, PhD, professor of kinesiology and health science at California State University, Fullerton, and co-director of the university's Center for Successful Aging. "When recovering from an illness, a person relies on amino acids. The less muscle tissue they have, the less of a reservoir there is."[29]

So if you get sick, having more stores of amino acids in your muscles gives you more building blocks to recover from illness. You have more fighting power in your bank account.

Feel better, reduce depression

Any exercise releases endorphins, those "feel good" hormones. Holistic psychiatrists now recommend exercise as one of the first steps to combat depression, Dr. Daniel Amen included. Dr. Amen takes a comprehensive holistic, life style approach to deal with depression and other psychiatric diseases. As he so eloquently teaches, the brain is an organ just like the heart, lungs, liver, and kidneys are organs. They all need healthy nutrition, exercise, and enough sleep to function optimally.[30]

Even your brain benefits from exercise

Male mice that exercised produced more mitochondria in their brains. The sedentary mice did not. Since mitochondria produce energy for the cell, the authors of this study commented, *"exercise training increases brain mitochondrial biogenesis, which may have important implications, not only with regard to fatigue, but also with respect to various central nervous system diseases and age-related dementia that are often characterized by mitochondrial dysfunction."*[31]

Improve sleep patterns

There's nothing like a good workout to help you sleep better.

Increase years of healthy living

Here's a wonderful surprise I discovered while researching the benefits of strength training. It decreases your chance of premature death due to a number of different diseases and specifically the chance of dying from cancer.[32] In this study the researchers followed 8762 men aged 20-80 years for almost 19 years. They measured muscle strength and consistently found that the stronger the muscles the less risk of dying of any cause including cancer, another great return on the investment of 15 minutes per week in SuperSlow™ weight strengthening.

You not only decrease your risk of premature death but also increase your ability to live in a healthy body for longer, a body that frees you to enjoy life, family, friends and activities you love. A healthy resilient body helps you fulfill your destiny on earth.

Did you ever imagine in your wildest dreams that with only 15 minutes of SuperSlow™ high intensity exercise per week you can create all of these benefits for your body?
Build Muscle Mass

- Increase fast twitch fibers
- Increase metabolism
- Increase metabolic efficiency

Counteract Metabolic Syndrome

- Lower blood sugars, even reversing diabetes 2
- Increase insulin sensitivity

Increase HGH levels
Lose fat faster
Builds Structural Integrity

- Increase muscle strength
- Retain strength in old age thereby reducing the risk of falls and broken bones
- Increase stamina
- Strengthen bones, even reversing osteoporosis
- Reduce lower back pain
- Improve joint movement increasing mobility
- Provide joint stability and protection
- Reduce symptoms of arthritis
- Improve balance

Strengthen heart

- Strengthen blood vessels
- Decrease high blood pressure
- Lowers your cholesterol LDL/HDL ratio
- Raise HDL cholesterol, the good cholesterol

Decrease oxidative stress and increase anti-oxidant production

- Increase lung volume
- Boost immunity

Create endorphins, which makes you feel better and reduces the risk of depression

- Improve sleep patterns
- Increase years of healthy living

Basically SuperSlow™ slows aging[33] [34] [35]
Live life abundantly!

CHAPTER 5
HEALTHY EATING PLAN

Despite Dr. McGuff's love for exercise, especially SuperSlow™, he agrees that eating healthy plays a greater role than exercise in becoming and staying healthy. Although he says it's difficult to put a percentage on the effects of eating versus exercise, eating healthy probably provides 70 to 80% of the benefits.

"You cannot exercise yourself out of a bad diet. You have to exercise with a good diet. You can have a good diet without exercise and still get fairly good results, but you cannot get good results with exercise and a bad diet."

Standard American Diet (SAD) highly inflammatory

"The standard American diet is highly inflammatory. It produces systemic inflammation of an order that is almost beyond belief. In that state, if you do exercise of any significant stress, you're just adding inflammation on top of the inflammation, and you're actually putting yourself at a bit of a risk."

Get Diet Straight First

"I advise people to get their diet straight, and then exercise. Because I think a highly inflammatory diet, in combination with the acute systemic inflammation that occurs as a part of the exercise stimulus, can actually be a negative thing."

"Diet and exercise are synergistic, they augment one another." Dr. McGuff quoted from interview with Dr. Mercola[36]

What is a good diet, a healthy eating plan?

The media presents us with so many different new diets every year that it's easy to get confused about how to eat. And many of these fad diets, even the ones embraced or created by main stream health care, have proven to have disastrous effects in the long term. In the early 1980s when I began to take an interest in healthy nutrition the debate was between Pritikin and Atkins. Pritikin advocated a very low fat diet and Atkins advocated a high-fat diet. So which was I to follow?

As I studied nutrition I came to realize that there's no one diet that fits everybody's unique metabolism. Atkins may actually work for some and Pritikin may actually work for some. However, over the years there have been some bleak results from following a very low fat diet. In a number of studies people with low levels of plasma omega-3 fatty acids experienced more depression.[37] One of the more drastic effects has been development of increased suicidal risk[38] in persons who had a very low serum cholesterol level.[39] Both the nervous tissues and every cell in the body need good fats and good cholesterol to function properly. Without good fats and cholesterol the body can't produce the sheaths that surround the nerves to protect them. A deficiency of these protective layers can lead to mental problems. Without good fats in their cell membranes cells cannot operate efficiently.

So usually there's a more middle of the road approach to eating healthy. My eyes were opened to the truth about nutrition when I became acquainted with the Price-Pottenger Nutrition Foundation (PPNF) and started studying the historical nutritional research material that the foundation is dedicated to preserving. One of these nutritional pioneers, Dr. Weston Price travelled around the world visiting five continents and 12 cultures in the 1930s. That was quite a fantastic accomplishment in those days without airplanes to get you around quickly. He had to travel by ship and ground transportation, except in Alaska where he had to fly in pontoon planes to reach remote people groups. Since he was a dentist he was interested in the underlying cause of tooth decay and gum disease in that part of the world where people ate the so called "modern diet" which consisted of a preponderance of white flour, white sugar, coffee and canned foods. So he decided to study native populations who were not exposed to those "products of trade".

The people in every culture he visited were exceptionally healthy when they were eating their native diet of whole fresh unadulterated food indigenous to their land. They cultivated, hunted or gathered their food right in their local region. Each culture had a source of animal protein, at least a few vegetables which they ate liberally, and a source of whole grain. Many of the cultures did not have access to fruit. Dr. Price thought that if he found a culture that also ate fruit they would be even healthier. However he discovered that the people who ate fruit were not any healthier than those who did not as long as they were eating whole native foods. These robust people had strong bones and teeth with wide dental arches. They were also very happy people and most of these cultures did not need doctors, dentists or policemen.

The story changed when they left their remote area to live in a city where they were exposed to the products of trade, white flour, sugar, coffee and canned goods. The first generation eating the "modern diet" developed severe tooth decay. If dentists were scarce, tooth decay led to very painful tooth abscesses that could even cause death. If the parents continued to eat the modern diet, the children born to them did not have the normal tribal facial features. Their jaws narrowed so teeth were crowded and crooked. Their mid-facial features narrowed too causing small sinuses and narrowed nostrils, a structural set up for sinus and breathing disorders. They too were susceptible to tooth decay and lessened immune response leading to more infections, or over-vigilant immune response leading to allergies and asthma.

Dr. Francis Pottenger, MD knew Dr. Price and studied his research. Practicing in southern California he said if he had the opportunity to coach parents to provide optimum nutrition to a child before he turned 18 years old he could help that child rebuild his body to the high level of health of Dr. Price's robust natives.

Dr. Melvin Page, another dentist interested in the underlying cause of dental disease continued the research of Dr. Price and Dr. Pottenger. Like the other two doctors he too discovered that the underlying causes of dental disease were the same as the underlying causes of degenerative diseases, the big killers of today, heart disease, diabetes and cancer.

Very sick people arrived at Dr. Page's clinic in Florida. He told them to eat meat, fish, eggs and vegetables and then checked their blood chemistry panel every few days. As their blood work came into balance eating the whole, healthy food they healed and went home healthy and invigorated.

Dr. Page and his associates developed more detailed instructions for following a healthy eating plan, a plan that incorporated the truth about which foods nourish the body well and allow it to stay in balance and which foods upset the body, knock it out of balance and cause disease. When I encountered Dr. Page's plan I knew I had found the truth about nutrition. My confusion about which diet to follow left. Now I look at a newly devised diet and compare it to the truth about nutrition as discovered by Drs. Price, Pottenger and Page. If it lines up with the truth, then I understand how it can help folks. If it doesn't, then buyer beware.

At the Page Clinic they tested the blood of hundreds of people before and after eating a food. If the food allowed the body chemistry to stay in balance, then that food served the body well. If it knocked the body chemistry out of balance, then it did not serve the body well. Some food knocked the body chemistry out of balance for a few hours, others for 12 to 24 or even 48 hours. By compiling all of this testing Dr. Page and associates developed a system of classifying food according to how it allowed the body to stay in balance or according to how it knocked the body out of balance. They also followed blood sugar levels after eating various foods and factored the fluctuations of blood sugar caused by food into their food classification chart.

Class A foods serve the body the best.

Can you guess what they are? If you said the same foods as Dr. Price's healthy natives ate you would be right. The Class A foods allow the body to stay in balance and include:

- Animal protein
- Vegetables
- Non-gluten grains

Class B foods are just a little harder to digest and fruit releases glucose into the blood faster during digestion:

- Fruit
- Nuts and seeds
- Whole grain, gluten containing

Class C foods:

- Dairy
- Citrus fruit
- Yeast, mushroom and mold containing food

Class D Sweeteners and Confections cause inflammation in the body and rob nutrients from the body:

- Anything sweet
- Any artificial sweetener

Class E Chemicals and Additives upset body chemistry:

- Any drug whether prescribed, over-the-counter or illicit
- Any man-made chemical or food additive
- Caffeine
- Tobacco
- Baking powder

So here's a simple way to think of food.

Choose most of your food for the day from the Class A list.
Eat a small amount of a variety of protein food such as beef or wild game, poultry, eggs, fish and other sea food. Vegetarians and vegans can choose a combination of beans, nuts, and grains as protein sources.

For general health's sake eat 5 servings of vegetables per day. One serving is about ½ cup. To stave off cancer, diabetes, heart disease and other killer diseases eat 7 servings of vegetables per day. You will age slower if you eat 10 servings of vegetables per day to prevent shortening of the telomeres at the end of your DNA each time they divide.

Eat a rainbow of colors of vegetables daily; green leafy, green, yellow-white, red-orange-purple, and root vegetables.

Each color group provides a different balance of vitamins, minerals and phytonutrients. So a rainbow of colors provides you a diversity of nutrients.

Non-gluten grains are easier to digest and less prone to cause allergy or digestive problems. Adventure into the taste and texture of brown rice, wild rice, teff, quinoa, amaranth and millet.

Choose some food from the Class B list.

Raw nuts and seeds keep you well-oiled with those healthy fats that your cells need.

Keep fruit to no more than 2 servings per day, preferably eaten away from your meals so they digest better. A serving size may be smaller than you would imagine; 1 small apple, 10 grapes, ½ banana. Always eat the whole fruit. Don't drink fruit juice due to its high concentration of sugar mostly in the form of fructose. And remember you don't have to eat fruit to be optimally healthy but they are refreshing and many contain high anti-oxidant levels.

If you tolerate the gluten grains and want to eat them, keep serving sizes small and eat only whole grains, not the white, processed kind. Gluten containing grains include wheat (and all of its cousins like spelt and kamut), rye and barley. Oats may be gluten-free if they are properly grown and processed.

Eat Class C foods if your body tolerates them and you want to eat them.

Citrus fruit may irritate the gastrointestinal tract in sensitive people. But if you tolerate it, then enjoy it. Eating the white part of the citrus fruit next to the outer coating gives you bioflavonoids that strengthen blood vessels and help allergies. If you tend to bruise easily be sure to eat that white part along with the juicy part.

Adults don't need to drink milk but cultured dairy products like yogurt and kefir provide good probiotics.

Avoid consuming Class D Sweeteners and Class E Chemicals which upset body chemistry and cause

inflammation in your tissues. Inflammation translates to pain and degeneration into disease.

Recently as I was buying a ticket to my granddaughter's basketball game, the lady selling the tickets said, "Are you Dr. Tillman?"

"Yes."

"And you teach about nutrition?"

"Yes."

Then she said, "I heard that eating sweets is like eating ground up glass. It tears up your insides. What do you think about that?"

"Hmm, I haven't heard that but it is a good way to visualize the inflammation and destruction of the human body brought about by eating sweets and other refined carbohydrates."

So if you're tempted (and most of us are addicted) to eat sweets, think of sweets as eating shards of glass that destroy your body slowly and subtly.

How many times per day should I eat?

The number of meals you eat per day can vary depending on where you are in healing your metabolism. If you're just beginning to switch from eating the Standard American Diet (SAD - but true) full of sweets and processed food to a healthy eating plan, then eating 5-6 small meals per day helps stabilize your blood sugar.

When you ate sweets frequently your blood sugar shot up dangerously high which sent emergency signals to your pancreas to squirt out more insulin to get that blood sugar down quickly. Because refined sweets absorb into the blood so quickly, suddenly you had no more sugar available in your GI tract when the insulin levels were high. So blood sugar levels plummeted leaving you shaky, irritable and craving more sweets. (Some symptoms of low blood sugar are more subtle occurring on a daily basis if you eat a lot of sweets.) If you obliged that sweet craving by grabbing another soda or candy bar or pastry, then your blood sugar shot up again. And thus the vicious cycle goes on and on.

Four major glands regulate blood sugar levels: your liver, pancreas, adrenals and thyroid gland. Those glands wear out from the wild blood sugar swings that occur multiple times per day when eating high-sugar foods. Worn out glands contribute to the development of the degenerative diseases that you want to avoid, the 3 big killer diseases of our culture; heart and blood vessel disease, diabetes and cancer.

Sweets poison your liver but it's such a subtle chronic poisoning that you don't even know it's happening. Sweets follow the same metabolic process as alcohol and can cause the same destruction to the liver that alcohol causes, a cirrhotic, scarred, unable to function liver. Without a liver you die! Worst of all this deadly liver process is occurring in some children very silently until it's too late and their liver function is dead. And it's all so preventable - just stop feeding them sweets, especially all of the processed foods containing high fructose corn syrup!

What's the solution to taming your blood sugar swings? Eat whole food containing some protein, complex carbohydrates and fat with each meal. As these whole foods digest they gradually drip glucose into your blood stream keeping your blood glucose at a steady healthy level. Your glands say, "Thank you for taking us out of that chronic emergency state that depletes us. We can function normally now."

Here's a couple of ways to easily prepare 5-6 small meals per day:

1. Choose a protein, a variety of colors of vegetables and a whole grain. Put them together as a stir-cook, soup, salad or stew. Prepare enough to feed you for the next 24 hours. Then divide it into 5 or 6 containers. Now your meals are ready to take wherever you go. When you're hungry eat one of those life-enhancing meals instead of grabbing that death-inducing doughnut.

Your meal may look like this: chicken, spinach, green snap peas, red peppers, onions, jicama and quinoa. Looks like a delicious salad to me or a great stir cook or even a wonderfully colorful soup. Use your imagination. Create your own delicious color combinations. If you need some help creating these delicious meals that's exactly what *Dr. Jo's Natural Healing Cookbook* does for you!

2. Or your meals could look like this:

- Breakfast: Eggs with veggies in an omelet or soft-boiled eggs and a bag of raw veggies for an on-the-go breakfast
- Mid-morning: 1 tablespoon pecans (omega-6 oils) and 1 tablespoon pumpkin seeds (omega-3 oils)
- Lunch: Beautiful Salad
- Mid-afternoon: same as mid-morning
- Dinner: Turkey, mashed potatoes and a colorful salad with avocado and a healthy dressing
- Before bed (if needed) a slice of that turkey

Keep some healthy food with you at all times so it's handy to eat when hunger crops up and so you don't resort to eating the death-inducing food that readily surrounds and entices us. I keep a bag of healthy nuts with me. Since it's important to eat a variety of oils I choose a nut that's high in omega-6 fatty acids and one that's high in omega-3 fatty acids, with a special emphasis on the omega-3 since most of us are so lacking in omega-3.

Healthy nuts and seeds, eat some daily with a special emphasis on the omega-3 category
Omega-6: almonds, pecans, sunflower seeds, sesame seeds
Omega-3: flaxseeds, pumpkinseeds, walnuts, fish, grass fed beef, eggs
Mono-saturated: Olive oil and olives, macadamia nuts, avocado

What about fruit?
Once those blood sugar swings settle down you can add some fruit to your eating plan. Be sure to eat only the whole fruit. Do not drink fruit juice which concentrates the sweets once again. Fruit contains the sugar fructose which stresses the liver. So limit your fruit to only 2 servings per day. And a serving size is smaller than you might think, one small apple, ½ banana, or 10 grapes. Whole fruit goes well with nuts as a between meal snack. Dr.

Page and colleagues counseled patients to avoid eating fruit the first 4-8 weeks on the healing diet to help heal their glands faster. That advice is very effective, but can be difficult to do. So it's better for you to eat a little fruit while healing your metabolism than to eat some sickeningly sweet food-like product such as candy, cake, cookies, pastry, doughnuts or sodas.

What proportion of protein, carbohydrate, and fat should I eat?

No wonder you're asking that question. The media assaults us all too frequently with the latest diet manipulations. One of the most devastating ones in the last ten years has been the brain washing about eating a low fat diet. We heard it from the lay press. We heard it from the medical establishment.

Now let's think about the percentage of protein-carbohydrate-fat allotment in our diets logically. You start with 100%. If you eat very low fat at only 10% what fills up the rest of the 100%? It has to be protein or carbohydrates. Think of this pie chart as your plate. If you only eat 10% of your calories from fat what would you add to your plate to compose the rest of the 100% of caloric intake? Let's say you eat 40% of your calories from protein. The carbohydrate then has to be the other 50%.

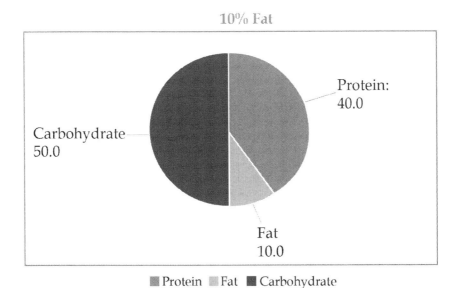

10% Fat

Protein: 40.0

Carbohydrate 50.0

Fat 10.0

■ Protein ■ Fat ■ Carbohydrate

When the low fat diet craze surfaced the processed food manufacturers faced this dilemma. The public now perceives fat as bad. So they thought, we have to find something that tastes good and appeals to them to take its place. What did they choose? Since proteins don't have a lot of taste appeal the food industry turned to carbohydrates in the form of very refined sugars and artificial sweeteners. But they knew consumers were very savvy. People were aware that sweets were not good for them either. So the food industry had to dream up another way to deceive us about the amount of sugar in a product.

Truth-in-labeling laws require companies to print the ingredients on the label in order, from the most abundant component to the least abundant component in their product. With the low fat craze they had to add lots of sweeteners to their breakfast or protein bars or cartons of yogurt. If they used all cane sugar it would have to be listed as the first and most abundant ingredient. Now they had a problem. If they printed the first component on the label as a sugar, consumers might realize that it wasn't the healthiest choice, that it was more like a candy bar than a nutrient dense healthy product. But the ingenuity of the industry solved that problem by adding several different sweeteners to the product. That's why you may see cane sugar, high-fructose corn syrup, dextrose, rice syrup solids and honey listed on the label of a product. Those sweeteners can now be scattered further down the list of ingredients on the package and you are deceived about the total content of sugar in the package. Never the less all of those various sweeteners add up to creating the same havoc in your metabolism.

So the low fat diet turned into a sugar overload for the American public. The liver of an adult can only handle about six to nine teaspoons of added sugars per 24 hours and the average American eats 22 teaspoons per day. One teaspoon of sugar equals 4 grams of sugar, helpful to know when reading food labels so you can calculate the number of teaspoons of sugar in a product.

We're killing our children, slowly and subtly

Dr. Robert Lustig, MD, pediatric endocrinologist at UCSF Medical School sees the devastation of this sugar overload in the children he treats. The switch to low fat processed food overloads their little bodies with sugar, more than their livers can handle. Children now suffer from adult diseases; obesity, Type 2 Diabetes, high blood pressure, cancer, early onset of hardening of the arteries and even non-alcoholic liver destruction because sugar is metabolized along the same pathways as alcohol. Have you ever watched your child's face turn pale white and pasty after eating a candy bar, cake or soda. That's a sure sign of sugar overload.

Sugar drives the development of the same inflammatory diseases in adults and adds dementia to the list.[40]

Can you see now how we get fooled when someone starts touting low fat diet or high fat diet or low carbohydrate diet or low protein diet? It's a manipulation that may drive a lot of sales of books, supplements and processed food but what does it do to our bodies? Probably not what all that hype promises. And worse, it can devastate our metabolism and drive us into an early onset of diseases of many types.

So let's get sensible and elaborate on that pie chart. Think of it as your dinner plate. You may have a metabolic type that thrives on eating equal amounts (in terms of calories) of protein, fat and carbohydrate. (One gram of fat contains 9 calories, whereas one gram of protein or carbohydrate contains 4 calories. So fats take up less room due to their higher caloric content per volume.)

Equal Amounts Protein Fat Carbohydrate

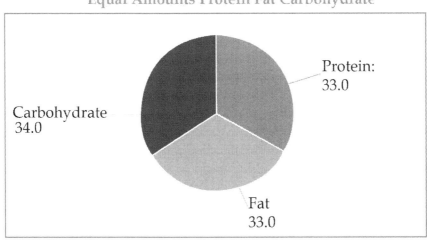

Protein ▨Fat ■Carbohydrate

Someone sitting at the table with you may have a metabolic type that thrives on eating a higher amount of healthy fat. Her pie chart could look like this:

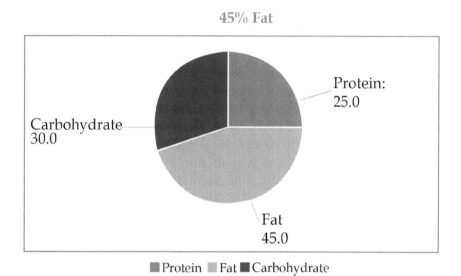

45% Fat

Protein:
25.0

Carbohydrate
30.0

Fat
45.0

■ Protein ▓ Fat ■ Carbohydrate

As I have touted for years, you are uniquely-you. Your metabolism is unique to you. The proportion of protein-fat-carbohydrate that you need is unique to you. Therefore one diet does not work for everyone. You need to experiment to see what works for you. When you stop eating sweets and the other addicting junk foods you can trust your body when it craves something, but only if you are eating healthy fresh whole food. The day you do your Fit in 15 workout you will probably feel the need to eat more protein. On a day when you do a lot of physical labor you may feel the urge to eat more carbohydrates. Sometimes fat may seem more satisfying. You can trust your body if you pay attention to it and eat only fresh whole foods.

As a starting point in finding the right ratio of protein-fat-carbohydrate that suits your uniquely-you body, try these proportions: protein 30%, fat 30%, carbohydrate 40%. Then vary the amount of each according to how you feel. Your chart would look like this:

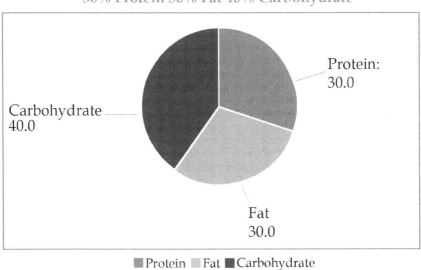

30% Protein 30% Fat 40% Carbohydrate

Protein:
30.0

Carbohydrate
40.0

Fat
30.0

▨Protein ▨Fat ■Carbohydrate

In actuality it's fairly easy to estimate the percentage of protein and carbohydrate on your plate but fat is a bit more difficult since it's intertwined with the other two. For more guidelines to get you started read Part 2 starting at page 49 of *Dr. Jo's Natural Healing Cookbook*.

Guidelines to Healthy Protein-Fat-Carbohydrate Sources:
Protein sources: poultry, eggs, fish, seafood, beef, lamb, pork
Healthy fat sources: nuts and seeds, coconut oil, avocado, olives, olive oil, butter from organically raised cows, grape seed oil
Complex carbohydrates: Vegetables including root vegetables, whole grains, legumes, and whole fruit

Avoid all refined carbohydrates because they devastate your body chemistry. Any whole food like sugarcane or whole wheat or a whole orange that's processed into its components becomes a refined food. In your thinking put a skull and cross-bones on them because that's what they are — poison — all concentrated sweets, white flour, fruit juices and anything made from them.

If you follow the eating plan in *Dr. Jo's Natural Healing Cookbook*, you don't need to worry at all about what not to eat.

Transition to eating 2 or at most 3 meals per day in a 12 hour period

After several months of eating 5-6 meals per day to stabilize your blood sugar and heal your metabolism consider transitioning to eating only 2-3 meals per day during a 12 hour period. Some doctors and scientists call this "intermittent fasting". With 12 hours to rest from processing food your body can turn its attention to healing, repair and detoxification. The overworked glands get to rest and regenerate. The blood sugar-insulin dysregulation comes into balance. The cells have a chance to repair and to dump stored toxins instead of always having to deal with the incoming substances.[41]

And perhaps best of all, your metabolism switches from sugar burning to fat burning. When you constantly feed yourself your body first utilizes the incoming glucose as fuel. When you give your body a break from food for a significant amount of time each 24-hour period then it mobilizes fat as fuel. That's what you want to be - a fat burner instead of a fat storer. The benefits are obvious for reaching your ideal weight and optimal state of health.

Going without food for 12 hours may seem daunting at first, but really it's as simple as not eating after 7 PM at night and waiting until 7 AM the next morning to eat breakfast. When you look at it that way it's not really that hard. You might even be able to stretch the fasting time out a little further, delaying breakfast until 8 or 9 AM. Some doctors think eating all of your meals in an 8 hour time period is even better for your health and metabolism. Since that's a bit harder to accomplish, aim for the 12-hour fasting time initially.

Intermittent fasting also boosts your human growth hormone (HGH) naturally, as much as 1300% in men and 2000% in women.[42] HGH helps you maintain and build your muscle mass and balance your metabolism. At the Intermountain Medical Center Heart Institute the cardiac researchers were surprised when the intermittent fasting participants' blood cholesterol levels increased, both the LDL and HDL components. Fortunately they realized that "Fasting causes hunger or stress. In response, the body releases more cholesterol, allowing it to utilize fat as a source of fuel, instead of glucose. This decreases the number of fat cells in the body," says Dr. Horne. "This is important because the fewer fat cells a body has, the less likely it will experience insulin resistance, or diabetes."

Other benefits of Intermittent fasting:

- Decrease in blood triglycerides
- Decreased blood pressure[43]
- Decrease in inflammation
- Modest decrease in fasting insulin and insulin resistance[44]

What time should I eat in relation to exercise?

Whether you eat before exercising depends on your current goals. If you want to lose weight, then fasting before exercise potentiates fat burning. Whenever you have less glucose in your blood you will shift to burning more fat. So if you want to lose 50 pounds, perform your high intensity exercise before breakfast for about 6 months. Or if you exercise later in the day wait at least 2 hours after a meal to exercise. Once you have reached your ideal weight, then shift to eating before you exercise to improve strength or speed.

Per Dr. Mercola:

"Intermittent Fasting and High-Intensity Exercise Is a Potent Combo for Weight Loss

When it comes to shedding unwanted pounds and reworking your fat-to-muscle ratio, high-intensity interval training (HIIT) combined with intermittent fasting is a winning combination that's hard to beat. When you combine these two strategies, especially if you exercise in a fasted state, it effectively forces your body to shed fat because your body's fat burning processes are activated by exercise and lack of food. The good news is that you don't have to keep on intermittently fasting forever if it doesn't appeal to you long-term. Also if you are already your ideal weight, then there really isn't much need to exercise fasting as it will limit your performance."[45] (Dr. Mercola)

If you exercise while fasting then it's very important to eat a recovery meal within 30 minutes of completion of the high intensity exercise to prevent brain and muscle damage. Fast-assimilating whey protein reaches your muscles within 10-15 minutes of swallowing it to provide amino acids for rebuilding the muscles. Ingesting 20 to 25 grams of a high quality whey protein right after your high intensity workout helps stimulate maximal increase in muscle mass.[46]

Participants in another study consumed their 20 grams of whey protein 30 minutes before their resistance training which increased their fat burning ability for 24 hours afterward.[47] So ingesting whey protein before a high intensity workout increases your metabolic rate which requires the burning of more fuel in the form of fat. That's the good news, getting rid of more fat. Perhaps ingesting 20 grams of whey protein before high intensity exercise and 20 grams afterward will give a double benefit of increasing fat burning and building muscle mass. Smaller sized people may need to decrease the whey protein to 10-15 grams before and after workouts.

So be very careful about what you eat in the 2-3 hours after your high intensity workout. Avoid eating any carbohydrates at all for at least two hours after your workout because they counteract the effects of the whey protein to build muscle and increase fat burning and specifically nullify the increased production of HGH. Carbs promote the release of somatostatin that shuts down the release of HGH. You surely don't want to miss out on the surge of HGH in the 2 hours following your workout. That 2 hour window gives you the benefits of a 2 hour cardio workout in relation to the amount of fat burned without the grueling assault on your body. For most of us this plan works the best for our metabolism and health. However, if you are an intense athlete in training, then carbohydrates after workouts help you recover faster. [48]

Avoiding carbohydrates before exercise is important as well to maintain the HGH release. Carbohydrates include sports drinks, fruit, pasta, root vegetables, grains, flour products, even starchy vegetables. Anything that's not protein or fat is a carbohydrate.

Once you reach your weight goal, then try eating before exercise to facilitate increasing your speed or strength. Personally I don't like to exercise immediately after eating because a large portion of blood diverts to the gastrointestinal tract to help digestion. Therefore, there's not as much blood to serve the muscles and they do not perform as well. However, waiting an hour or so after a meal when the food has digested and nutrients are entering the blood stream serves the muscles well. At this point they get more blood and more fuel to facilitate good performance.

Since we need to avoid carbohydrates before and after high intensity exercise, drinking 15-20 grams of a high quality whey protein 30 minutes before exercise and another 15-20 grams within 30 minutes after exercise appears to provide the very best benefits in increasing muscle mass, increasing HGH and decreasing fat cells. Since most of us perform Fit in 15 only once per week that amount of protein should not overload our systems.

What qualifies as a healthy whey protein? Only buy whey protein that comes from grass-fed, organically raised cows free of injected hormones and pesticides. Be sure the whey is produced by cold processing without acid treatment which protects the valuable immunoglobulins and lactoferrins. Whey protein derived from pasteurized milk or other heat treatments damage the protein in the whey making it difficult to digest and toxic to your body. Also avoid any products with added sweeteners, especially artificial sweeteners. Permissible sweeteners include stevia or Lo-Han, a non-glycemic fruit sweetener. I buy a non-sweetened whey protein and add my own stevia if needed. Check to be sure the label says "whey protein concentrate", not whey protein isolates and look for medium chain fatty acids, not long-chain fatty acids which are harder to digest.[49] Currently I buy Designs for Health Whey Cool protein powder. You can find it with an Internet search. Dr. Mercola also sells an excellent whey protein at www.mercola.com.

Synopsis of the Healthy Eating Plan

On the day you perform your Fit in 15 workout (or other High Intensity Interval Training - HIIT)
After an overnight or at least a 2 hour fast:
Consume 15 to 20 grams of high quality whey protein before your workout.*

Consume another 15-20 grams of high quality whey protein after your workout. A smaller person may need to decrease the amount of protein intake, perhaps 10-15 grams before and after the workout.

Do not eat any carbohydrates for at least 2 hours before and after your workout. Eating carbohydrates 2 hours before or less than 2 hours after your workout shuts down the HGH production. You certainly want to maintain this benefit of your intense efforts.

*If you are in the phase of losing weight, then do not consume the whey protein before your workout.

In the phase of stabilizing your metabolism after converting to the Healthy Eating Plan:
Eat 5 to 6 small meals per day consisting of a variety of colors of vegetables, high quality protein sources, nuts and seeds, whole grains (non-gluten may be best) and no more than 2 small servings of fruit per day.

Continue eating 5-6 small meals per day for 4 to 8 weeks. When you are ready to transition to eating only 2-3 meals per day, gradually start spacing your meals farther apart.

Convert to fat-burner instead of a sugar burner

Fast for 12 hours per day by eating your meals within a 12 hour time frame daily. Continue to choose your food from colorful vegetables, healthy proteins, nuts and seeds, whole grains (non-gluten may be best) and no more than 2 small servings of fruit per day.

If you eat your last bite of food at 7 PM then wait until 7 AM or after to eat your next meal.

Fasting for more than 12 hours (even up to 16 hours) may be even more beneficial for your metabolism. Listen to your body and determine what works best for your uniquely-you metabolism.

CHAPTER 6
HIGH INTENSITY INTERVAL TRAINING

Fit-in-15 (SuperSlow™) - 15 minutes per week - that's all you need to do to stay fit.

If you want to learn a little more about another high intensity workout, then read on. If not you can stop reading here.

Fifteen minutes of Fit-in-15 training per week keeps us at a great fitness level. Once I've done my workout I figure I've done all I really need to do for the rest of the week in regard to keeping fit. But I like to move! My muscles yell at me if I just sit around. So I like to keep active doing things I enjoy like gardening, walking, hiking or doing the "have-to" list of chores like housekeeping. Some days I like to sprint while jogging or swimming in the pattern called High Intensity Interval Training, HIIT.

A conceptually simple exercise HIIT only takes around 15-20 minutes per session. This time you exercise intensely by moving through space. You can apply HIIT to any exercise that you enjoy like bicycling, swimming, dancing, using the elliptical trainer, etc.

The Exercise

- Short periods of exertion reaching 80-95% of maximal heart rate[50]
- Followed by short periods of rest slowing to 40-50% of maximal heart rate
- Repeat 7 to 9 times
- Examples:
    Walk 30 seconds fast, rest 45 seconds or more
    Bike as fast and hard as you can for 30 seconds, rest 30-60 seconds.
    Swim 30 seconds intensely, rest 60 seconds or more

Let's review a swim HIIT pattern. Warm up for about 5 minutes before entering the intensity cycle. Slowly swim a few laps until you feel warmed up. Cycle 1: swim as hard and fast as you possibly can until you're gasping for breath for about 30 seconds. You want to try to reach 80-95% of your maximal heart rate in the intensity part of the exercise. Then rest for 30 to 60 seconds or more until your heart rate comes down and you are breathing comfortably again. That completes the first cycle. Repeat this cycle for 6-7 more times. Then cool down with a few more easy laps.

Phil Campbell states:

"There are many different ways you could do...HIIT as long as you can get totally exhausted in 30 seconds or less. That's the key. If you can't go longer than 30 seconds [because you are so exhausted]-no matter if you are a professional athlete or just starting - that means you're doing it correctly. It has to be so intense that [before the] 30 seconds [are over], you're just praying for those last seconds to go by..."[51]

In other words if you become totally exhausted in 30 seconds or less, you're performing the intense interval correctly. It feels "very hard". You have difficulty talking to someone.

Follow a similar pattern in walking.

- Warm up for 5 minutes or so
- Walk as fast as possible for 15-30 seconds
- Rest for 30-60 seconds until you breathe comfortably again
- Repeat the cycle 6-8 more times.

Keep Exercise Interval Short

- 30 seconds is enough
- Then concentrate on recovery
  Calm your mind
  Picture your heart rate slowing down
  Each time you exhale, see your heart rate slowing down
  When your heart rate recovers, do another intense interval

Various trainers and coaches advocate different lengths for the intense intervals and different lengths for the recovery phase. The intense interval ranges from 20 to 60 seconds and the rest phase from 10 seconds to 4 minutes.[52] For most of us the 30 second maximum interval works well and you can choose the number of minutes for your rest phase.

Apply this intensity-rest pattern of exercise to any exercise you like. If you bicycle in steep terrain it may be harder to apply since the uphills and downhills require different intensities of effort. In the winter when we can't bike outside we put our bikes up on training stands. That way we can set the resistance and get a good HIIT workout. When the sun comes out and dries up all the rain (and snow) we're in shape to bike outdoors again.

Exercise beginners:

Always check with your doctor before starting an exercise program!

If you have a family history of coronary artery disease, smoke cigarettes, have hypertension, diabetes (or pre-diabetes), abnormal cholesterol levels or obesity you can be at increased risk for heart damage with intense exertion. You must get clearance from your doctor before starting HIIT or Fit-in-15. Your doctor may direct you to start with an exercise program closely supervised by trained medical personnel before you can graduate to Fit-in-15 or HIIT.

The American College of Sports Medicine makes these recommendations before starting an exercise program:

"The First Step Before you begin an exercise program, take a fitness test, or substantially increase your level of activity, make sure to answer the following questions. This physical activity readiness questionnaire (PAR-Q) will help determine if you're ready to begin an exercise routine or program.

Has your doctor ever said that you have a heart condition or that you should participate in physical activity only as recommended by a doctor?

Do you feel pain in your chest during physical activity?

In the past month, have you had chest pain when you were not doing physical activity?

Do you lose your balance from dizziness? Do you ever lose consciousness?

Do you have a bone or joint problem that could be made worse by a change in your physical activity?

Is your doctor currently prescribing drugs for your blood pressure or a heart condition?

Do you know of any reason you should not participate in physical activity?

If you answered yes to one or more questions, if you are over 40 years of age and have recently been inactive, or if you are concerned about your health, consult a physician before taking a fitness test or substantially increasing your physical activity. If you answered no to each question, then it's likely that you can safely begin exercise."[53]

Once you are cleared by your doctor, be cautious in starting an intense exercise program. Take your time to build up. It's a process. Consider starting with Fit-in-15 to build your muscle mass and cardiovascular reserves. Then if you want to try some HIIT, start with short intervals and gradually increase them in subsequent workout sessions. Your workouts might look like this:

- Week 1
  Interval—15 seconds
  Rest - 2 minutes
  Repeat 4-5 times

- Week 2
  Interval—17 seconds
  Rest - 2 minutes
  Repeat 4-5 times

- Week 3
  Interval—20 seconds
  Rest - 2 minutes
  Repeat 4-5 times

- Week 4
  Interval—25 seconds
  Rest - 2 minutes
  Repeat 5-6 times

- Week 5
    Interval—30 seconds
    Rest - 2 minutes
    Repeat 5-6 times

- Week 6
    Interval—30 seconds
    Rest - 1.5 minutes
    Repeat 5-6 times

- Week 7
    Interval—30 seconds
    Rest - 1.5 minutes
    Repeat 6-7 times

- Week 8
    Interval—30 seconds
    Rest - 1.5 minutes
    Repeat 6-7 times

Continue to progressively adjust your uniquely-you program. Find your level of safety. Don't try to keep up with anyone else. It's not a competition.

Pay attention to how your body responds to this type of high intensity training. Use your ingenuity to gradually increase the length of the interval and decrease the length of the rest period. But give yourself plenty of time to fully recover before performing the next intense interval effort.

The rest time can be longer and still give you the same cardiovascular and conditioning benefits. The number and intensity of the peak exertional efforts create the improvement in your fitness level. In several research studies the rest period was 4 to 4.5 minutes with only 30 seconds of intense effort repeated 3 to 5 times. The participants still achieved remarkable improvements in their fitness levels. Isn't it great to know that more time spent in exercise is not better? With short periods of intense effort we can accomplish more for our fitness level and throw guilt out the window. That feeling of having to do more or never being able to exercise enough goes bye-bye.[54]

In one particularly interesting study the participants gained dramatic improvement in exercise performance in a 2 week period with only 15 minutes of intense exercise total. But that intense exercise was broken into 30 second sprints. Sixteen volunteers from the student population of McMaster University participated. Six men and 2 women participated in the training program. Eight other men were in the control group that did not train. They were all recreationally active people enjoying jogging, cycling, aerobics, etc. two to three times per week but they were not participating in a structured training program.

Both groups became familiar with testing methods and training devices before they underwent testing and did a practice ride. Then at two separate times they cycled as long and hard as they could until they were completely fatigued (endurance test = endurance time to fatigue) on an electronically braked cycle ergometer. The control group then went about their usual daily activities for 2 weeks. The study group participated in six training sessions total, one on Monday, Wednesday and Friday for 2 weeks. In each session they sprinted "all-out" for 30 seconds 4 to 7 times with 4 minutes recovery time. The number of 30-second sprints increased from 4 to 7 per session over the first 5 sessions. For the last session they completed four 30-second sprints.[55]

At the end of the two weeks both groups again cycled through an endurance test to fatigue. The study group **"doubled endurance capacity during cycling exercise"** from 26 min to 51 min cycling at 80% of pre-training VO2 peak (peak oxygen consumption) - after only six HIT sessions. The control group's endurance remained the same as the pre-test level with no improvement.[56] (Some researchers shorten HIIT to HIT by hyphenating the Intensity-Interval portion to High Intensity-Interval Training.)

Doubling endurance with only 15 minutes total of intense effort (spread over 2 weeks though) is dramatically remarkable. Doesn't it get you excited about expending that intense energy to get those kinds of gains? Seems a lot better than the long slow stuff that eats up a lot of time and does not deliver those remarkable gains in exercise fitness.

Before you start HIIT, remember that these folks were young and already actively exercising. Use some precaution in starting your program.

Precautions

Fit-in-15 versus HIIT, which is best?

For overall fitness development and safety, I prefer Fit-in-15 over HIIT as my main training program.

More stressful on musculoskeletal system

Most HIIT exercise places more stress on the joints and more wear and tear on the muscles and bones. With Fit-in-15 there's a built in governor that keeps you from stressing your joints and overstressing your muscles. Since you can only lift a certain amount of weight determined by your muscle mass and strength at the moment, you won't be jerking heavier weights which could damage joints and muscles. Also the smooth slow nature of the movement through the weight lifting exercise adds another layer of protection.

Swimming intense intervals in HIIT tends to spare the joint and bone trauma, but most other HIIT choices cause a lot of impact on the musculoskeletal system as in jump roping, dancing, and running. Stationary bicycling and using the elliptical machine may fall somewhere in between.

Fit-in-15 increases muscle mass much faster and more efficiently than HIIT. Therefore you achieve the benefits explained in Chapter 4 more rapidly.

Beginners beware of running sprints, outside or on treadmill

Unless you are a very experienced runner avoid running as your first entry exercise into HIIT because of uneven terrain that may cause a fall and because of the high impact on your joints and muscles.

The same advice goes for running on a treadmill. Becoming accustomed to that moving belt takes time and it's easy to feel off balance. Once you're down you're whisked right off the end of the treadmill.

Achieving the intensity level may be harder

When you first begin High Intensity Interval Training your muscles may not be strong enough to push you into that intense effort required to accomplish an effective interval effort. Therefore achieving an optimal fitness level may take longer than Fit-in-15 takes.

On the other hand, once you become more fit with HIIT and your cardiovascular and lung systems gain a lot of reserve you may hit a plateau where you can't run fast enough or swim fast enough to reach that maximal level needed to keep increasing your fitness level.

Highly Trained Athletes

For athletes who are already highly trained "improvements in endurance performance can be achieved **only** through high-intensity interval training (HIIT)."[57] If you enjoy endurance sports these researchers claim that once you achieve a high level of endurance fitness, the only way to break through to the next level of endurance is to engage in HIIT. And for those of us who just like to stay fit HIIT and Fit-in-15 can increase our endurance if we just want to go out and run or bike or cross-country ski. HIIT and Fit-in-15 sound like a win-win situation to me.

Summary

Because Fit-in-15 so effectively builds muscle mass and strength and builds in all of its many other benefits rapidly, I choose it as my primary exercise mode. It's quick (15 minutes per week). I can do it at home with only a little bit of equipment (some weights) and it doesn't cost anything on a weekly basis. But most of all it's just the best exercise program to build fitness and stay healthy.

Then there are the times that I feel like moving through space and getting my blood circulating faster. So I swim intense intervals or bike intervals on my stationary bike.

Because I ran (never very fast) when I was training for the sprint triathlon, I'm accustomed to running so sometimes I enjoy running intervals too.

Keep in mind that it can take a full week or even more for your muscles to completely recover and rebuild after a Fit-in-15 workout. Performing another intense exercise can interfere with that muscle recovery process. So you may not gain anything and you could lose muscle mass by combining Fit-in-15 and HIIT in the same week. Dr. McGuff recommends avoiding any other intense exercise for at least 2 days before and 2 days after SuperSlow™.

Whatever exercise you choose, have fun!

CHAPTER 7
KEEP MOVING—NO COUCH POTATOES

You feel good! You've finished your 15 minutes of intense Fit-in-15 exercise and you're ready to lie on the couch for the rest of the week.

But HOLD ON - NO - that's not the way it works. Sitting for just an hour can undo all that great effort you invested in your health improvement. Bummer you say. No, not bummer, now you're ready to have fun keeping your body supple and moving regularly because the hard work is over.

Seriously, numerous studies linked prolonged sitting to increased risk of developing diabetes, heart disease and death from a variety of other causes. Those who sit the most have a 147% increase in the relative risk for developing heart and blood vessel disease and 112% relative risk increase for developing diabetes. Sitting also contributes to the development of Alzheimer's disease.[58] Sitting for 8 hours increased the risk of developing diabetes for men by 90%. Sitting elevates blood pressure, blood sugar, cholesterol and toxic build up in your body.

Sitting increases the risk of dying from any cause by 50%, a risk as great as that of smoking.[59]

Who would have thought that sitting is as dangerous as smoking cigarettes? "Sitting is the new smoking." But let's think about that a minute. How much time do we spend sitting every day? Dr. James Levine, M.D., Ph.D. is the Director of the Mayo Clinic/Arizona State University Solutions Initiative and the inventor of the treadmill desk. In 1995 he started "the Active Life Research Team, a research program that would become the most comprehensive, data-rich study on nutrition, activity and behavior related to weight management and obesity prevention ever undertaken, sponsored by the National Institute of Health."[60] They now alert us to the consequences of prolonged sitting, proclaiming that our sedentary lifestyle is the greatest factor in the increasing obesity crisis. But let's keep the overall picture in perspective. Data certainly shows that sitting too much causes physiologic problems that contribute to obesity and degenerative diseases. However, most problems have multiple causes that produce the bad results. Sitting is one of those causes.

Another researcher, Dr. Joan Vernikos, previously studied the rapid decline of astronaut's bodies in a weightless environment in her position at NASA. Prior to entering weightlessness astronauts were more fit than most people but without the force of gravity their bodies deteriorated rapidly to that of an elderly person. She then turned her research to examine the effects of prolonged sitting and found the effects similar to those that developed in the astronauts. Her remedy includes performing a great variety of movements 36 times during the day that resist gravity. "Dr. Vernikos recommends "playing" with gravity and becoming inventive: stooping, squatting, reaching, bending, stretching, jumping, etc. She has various suggestions for incorporating more movement into your life in her book, *Sitting Kills, Movement Heals.*"[61]

When we lived on farms and ranches we moved about all day, keeping our physiological processes revved up most of the time. Farmers and ranchers don't have much time to sit in their busy active days. They sit just long enough to rest a bit, about 3 hours per day total.

The average American sits 10 to 15 hours per day and if we sleep 8 hours per 24 hours (that's a good health habit), that only leaves 1 to 6 hours for moving around. We sit at work, in front of a computer, video game or TV and in the car. We are slaves to the chair. According to Dr. Levine whenever we sit important processes come to a halt in our cells. But when we stand up and get moving again, they're reactivated.

Your body says, "Oh the muscles are moving again. We've got to get busy supplying them with more blood flow to deliver oxygen and nutrients so they can keep moving." The blood glucose starts moving into the muscle cells to be turned into energy. That stabilizes blood sugar and insulin levels. The cells also step-up the processing of triglycerides (blood fats) and cholesterol which contributes to healthy homeostasis in the body. All of these mechanisms burn more calories and foster healthy physiological processes in your body.

Sitting shuts off those healthy activities again.

But what about work and school? We immediately start saying, "I have to sit at work. I have to sit at school". Dr. Levine addressed those problems too, especially in the work place. He invented the desk treadmill. It should be interesting to try that out. Can you walk and chew gum at the same time? Or can you walk and type at the same time? What a great challenge.

Others designed standing desks for the work place. But then isn't standing for prolonged times hard on the body too? Well, yes, it could be, but we naturally shift from one foot to the other, sway and fidget when we stand. All those motions keep the cells on alert to keep those healthy physiological processes activated. If we're already standing up, why not walk over to a colleague's desk instead of sending an email?[62]

Company executives may be won over to the standing desk and encouraging employees to move more during the day when they realize that movement increases productivity and creativity. Instead of sitting at meetings several hours per day participants will take walks to discuss their agendas, move around the office more and be cognizant of staying off their bottoms as much as possible by utilizing standing desks and possibly even the treadmill desk. Maybe those folks that hang out at the water cooler in the office aren't as lazy and under productive as we thought since walking around sparks creativity and increases efficiency.

Have you ever experienced a sudden flood of creativity flowing after exercising or taking an enjoyable walk outside? When on vacation on the beautiful California coast, I returned to camp after a refreshing jog down the coastline and immediately dictated most of my cookbook. The inspiration flowed. Similar moments of inspiration and creativity opened up when biking. I began to think that I should carry a device that takes dictation when I'm out moving about in nature. Similarly, blessing employees with the gift of moving about can increase the company's creativity and productivity.

Children innately know that it's not good to sit but they have trouble convincing the teachers of that. So we train the moving-about out of them. Of course we don't want chaos in the classroom but perhaps as teachers engage in more moving-about they will become inspired in ways they can allow children to move more as well. Perhaps standing desks will become part of classrooms. Some teachers have allowed certain students to sit at their desks on exercise balls which of necessity stimulates more movement to maintain balance. Sitting on exercise balls instead of chairs might be a good option for adults too.

Sometimes I feel like a kid again. I just cannot sit still for hours tied to a desk. Despite loving to write, the discomfort of sitting for hours at the desk overcomes me and I have to jump up and do something else. I always feel better physically when I am very active in the garden or out on the property tending our trees and controlling brush and weeds. My mind feels brighter and more joyful, my gut feels happier and my muscles and joints feel more supple and comfortable. I can't imagine how I would tolerate sitting for hours and hours again in lectures in the first couple of years of medical school. What a relief to find out that sitting for a long time is detrimental to health. Now I purposely try to break up the sitting, writing for a while by getting up and working outside, or catching up on some housework or taking a walk.

How do we increase activity in our daily living?

Use your imagination. Let's get creative.

Dr. Levine says to sit no more than 50 minutes per hour and to move about no less than 10 minutes per hour. Maybe as we sit at our desks we could set a timer for 50 minutes to remind us to move it!

Dr. Vernikos says to set a timer for every 15 minutes and get up and move it.

Walk down the hallway or outside exaggerating your arm and leg swings. That cross-crawl type of movement helps center and stimulate your brain as well as stimulate your muscles.

If you don't look too goofy to folks in your surroundings stand up and walk in place lifting your knees until your thighs are parallel to the floor. With each leg movement tap the top of your thigh with your opposite hand (right hand to left knee; left hand to right knee).

Stand up and move around while talking on the phone.

Stand up while eating lunch. Go outside to eat if you can to get some healthy sunshine.

Walk over to your colleague's space to toss around an idea instead of calling or emailing.

Take a walk to discuss options in meetings of a small group of people instead of sitting in a conference room.

Work at a stand-up desk.

Try sitting on an exercise ball when sitting at your desk. You'll probably find you have to move a bit to keep your balance.

Stand up and swing your body from side to side letting your arms flow with the swing and your eyes track with the swing. Your eyes need a rest too.

Stand up and look as far away as you can frequently to rest your eyes.

Try reading documents or books standing up and moving a bit.

Incorporate Dr. Vernikos' suggestions of stooping, squatting, reaching, bending, stretching and jumping but be aware of what your joints can tolerate.

Find a parking space a distance from your destination to help you take more steps during the day.

Take the stairs instead of the elevator. Now that's a gravity-defying exercise when going upstairs.

Any added steps during the day help to keep you healthier. Challenge yourself to find ways to walk more every day, not long walks, just extra steps interspersed in your daily routines.

Have you ever walked downstairs to get something and then don't remember why you went downstairs? Once you get back upstairs you suddenly remember what it was and trot back downstairs? Now I don't have to feel inefficient when I do that. I just chalk it up to extra steps that keep me healthier.

Maybe we should throw the remote control for the TV away. Channel surfer guys you would get a lot more exercise getting out of your recliner to change the channels.

And popping up off the couch during commercials - great idea.

Try watching some TV standing up.

Or sit on an exercise ball while watching TV. Actually our grandkids teach us how to be very active while watching TV. They constantly bounce while sitting on the ball, flip over on their stomachs and roll back and forth or take a flying roll across the ball onto the couch. Kids innately know how to stay healthy with activity.

While sitting in a car, pump your feet up and down periodically. Squeeze your other muscles. Turn your head from side to side. Keep those muscles on alert. Drivers can do some of the same movements when it's safe to do so.

Performing a few stretch movements between episodes of sitting may be an option too.

Stretching

The role of stretching can be a controversial subject. Dr. McGuff in *Body by Science* explains that athletes who stretch before a workout or athletic event decrease the power in their muscles and impair their performances. He goes on to explain that stretching after SuperSlow™ decreases the ability of the muscle to maximally improve strength in the regeneration phase. He also says that adults are not meant to be as flexible as children because adult bones have grown to occupy more of the joint space. Forced stretching in adulthood can damage the joints. According to Dr. McGuff the range of joint movements used in the SuperSlow™ exercises induce the appropriate amount of flexibility around the joints.

I respect Dr. McGuff's research and his in-depth knowledge about the physiology of strengthening muscles. Therefore I honor what he says about stretching. However, I still feel better if I perform some stretching exercises without overstretching muscles and ligaments.

My solution: Engage in stretching a day or two after my Fit-in-15 workout.

One idea: intersperse a few stretches to break up your hours tied to the chair.

Fitness experts, sports trainers, doctors, etc. recommend lots of different ways to stretch and lots of different stretching positions. Variety is the spice of life so if you like adventure do some research and find the stretches you like best. In the following pages you can review some simple stretches that Dr. Jo likes, starting at the top of the body and proceeding downward, an easy to remember routine.

Then there are the questions about how to stretch, what to stretch, how long to hold a stretch and how often to stretch. A bounty of research comes up with a variety of conclusions and differences for younger folks and seniors, for instance younger people seem to gain maximal benefit by holding a stretch for 30 seconds, whereas seniors take longer at 60 seconds. The following guidelines encompass the majority opinion on safe and effective stretching principles.

First employ these basic principles of stretching to improve flexibility and prevent damage to joints and ligaments:

1. Only stretch muscles. Avoid placing joints into positions of abnormal function. For example, do not put your knee in a position that stretches it side to side. Doing so could stretch the ligaments and destabilize the knee joint.
2. Warm up for 4-5 minutes before stretching. If you sit at a desk for long hours, take a walk down the hall or better yet, outside before stretching. Or just march in place touching your right hand to your left knee, left hand to

your right knee. Another great warm-up option: swing your torso turning slowly to the right and left relaxes your whole body and your eyes. Let your arms hang loose and follow the swing naturally. And allow your eyes to relax and follow the turn of your head.

3. Stretch until you just feel tension but not pain. Stretching in pain initiates a protective reflex in the muscle so it contracts, thus defeating your purpose in stretching.

4. Hold the stretch for at least 30 seconds but not more than 60 seconds. As the muscle relaxes you may be able to increase the length a fraction of an inch as you hold the stretch. Stretching more than 60 seconds can actually damage tissues.

5. Stretch each muscle 1 to 3 times per week for 30 to 60 seconds.[63]

6. Most of these stretches are performed in a standing position so you can do them just about anywhere. The last 4 are performed on the floor or other firm surface. If the floor is too firm for you, perform them on an exercise mat.

Enjoy A Set of Simple Stretches
on the following pages

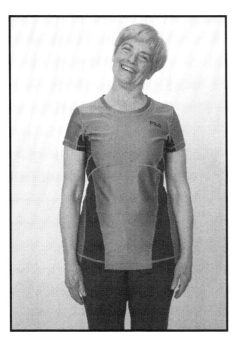

Neck Stretches

Lean your head toward your right shoulder until you feel a slight tension. Hold for 30-60 seconds and return to head neutral position.

Repeat leaning your head toward your left shoulder.

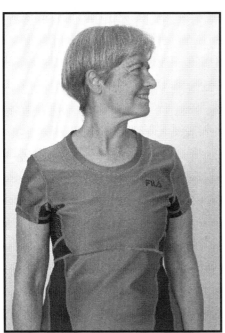

Rotate your head toward your right shoulder until you feel a slight tension. Hold for 30-60 seconds and return to head neutral position.

Repeat rotating your head toward your left shoulder.

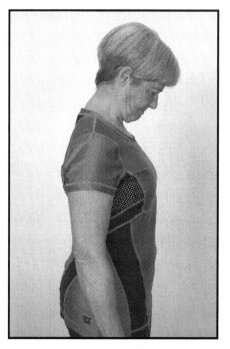

Touch your chin to your chest. Hold for 30 to 60 seconds. Return to head neutral.

Arm and Shoulder Stretches

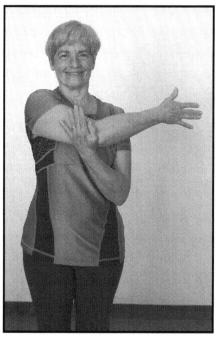

Move your right arm across your chest with elbow slightly bent. Place your left hand on your right arm just above the right elbow. Apply just enough pressure to feel the stretch in the shoulder without causing pain. Hold for 30 to 60 seconds. Repeat with left arm across chest.

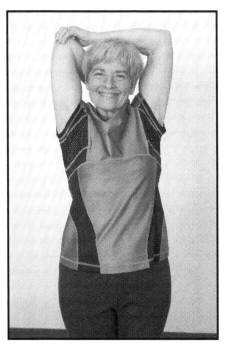

Raise your right arm straight up. Then bend at the elbow so your right hand is on your upper back. With your left hand grasp your right elbow and pull your right arm gently backwards until you feel the stretch in your right triceps muscles. Hold for 30 to 60 seconds.

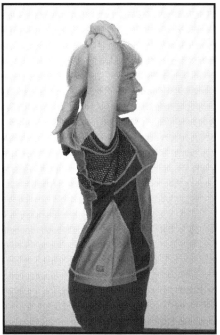

Repeat this stretch with your left arm.

Side view of the triceps stretch.

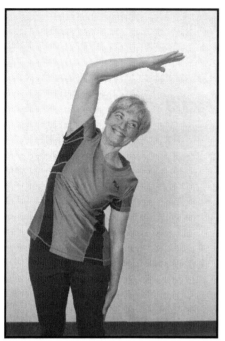

Torso Stretch

Raise your right arm straight up then bend your elbow so your forearm is over your head. Lean to the left until you feel the stretch in your right torso. Hold for 30 to 60 seconds.

Repeat for your left side.

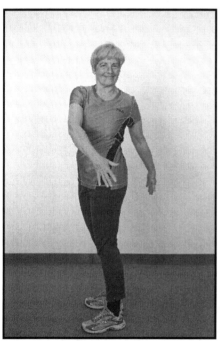

Torso Twist

Twist your body to the left at your waist with your arm leading the twist. Hold for 30 to 60 seconds.

Repeat this twist in the opposite direction.

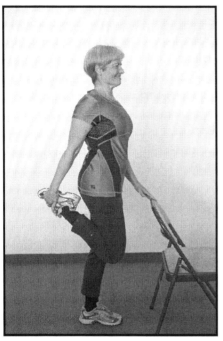

Quadriceps Stretch

Stand straight. Hold onto a chair or other stable object to balance yourself. Bend your right leg and grasp your foot with your right hand. Pull gently until you feel the stretch in the quadriceps muscles (the front of your thigh). Hold for 30 to 60 seconds.

Repeat for the left quadriceps muscles.

When you are strengthened adequately to balance on one leg, instead of holding onto a chair, raise your opposite arm straight up while holding the quad stretch. You get the added bonus of improving your balance.

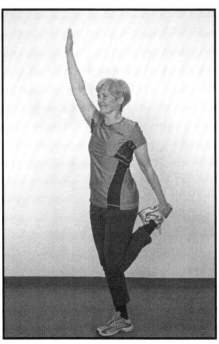

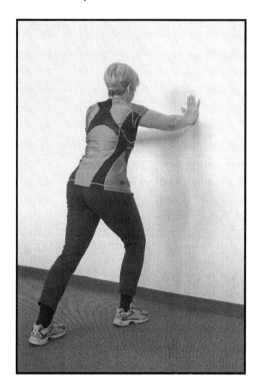

Calf Stretch
Place your hands on a wall about shoulder width apart. Keep both feet pointed forward.

Step back with your left foot keeping your left heel on the ground and your knee only slightly bent. Leave your right foot closer to the wall.

Lean into wall with your hips until you feel a stretch in the calf of the extended left leg.

Hold for 30 to 60 seconds.

Repeat with left leg.

To increase the stretch, move your foot farther back.

To stretch the Achilles tendon bend your knee in the same position and lower your hips.

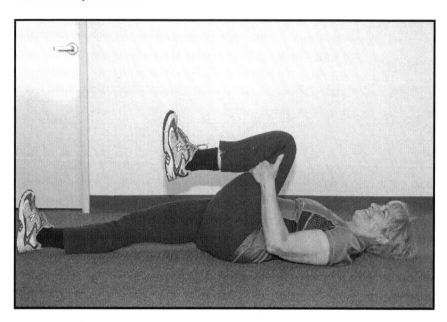

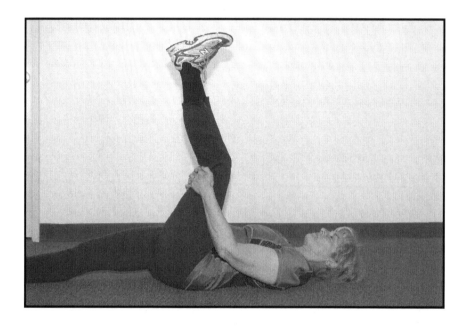

Gluteus and Lower Back Stretch

Lay flat on your back. Bend at your left knee and pull your knee towards your chest. Place both hands on the posterior thigh just below the knee. Pull gently toward your chest until you feel the stretch in your gluteus muscles (buttocks). Hold for 30 to 60 seconds.

Repeat on right side.

Hamstring Stretch

Lay flat on your back on a firm surface. Lift your left leg straight up with the knee only slightly bent. Place both hands on your posterior thigh just below your knee. Pull gently toward your chest until you feel the stretch in the hamstring muscles on the back of your thigh. Hold 30 to 60 seconds.

Repeat on the right side.

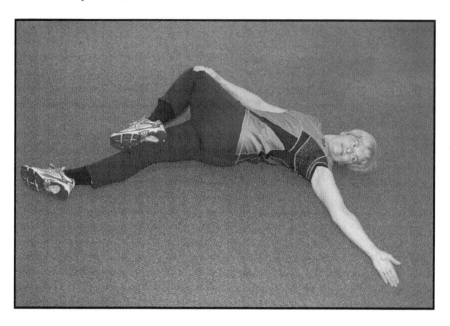

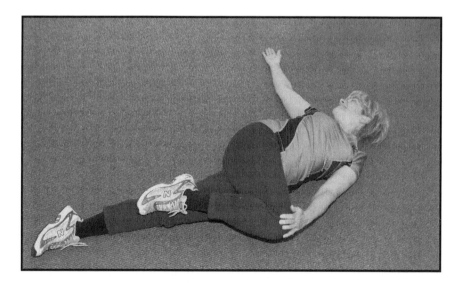

Lower Back and Side of Hip Stretch
Lay on your back on a firm surface. Bend your left knee and place your left leg across your body.

Stretch your left arm out perpendicular to your body and turn your head to look at your left hand. Your torso will now be mildly twisted.

Place your right hand on the outside of your left knee and gently press your bent knee toward the floor until you feel the gentle stretch in your lower back and side of hip.

Keep both shoulders on the floor. Keep feet and ankles relaxed.

Hold stretch for 30 to 60 seconds.

Repeat with right leg flexed and crossed over the body.

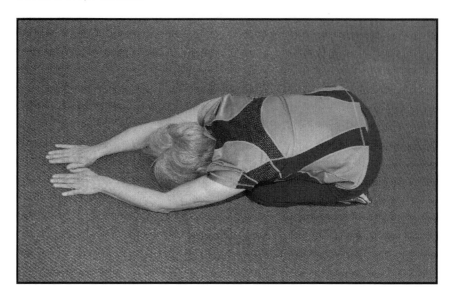

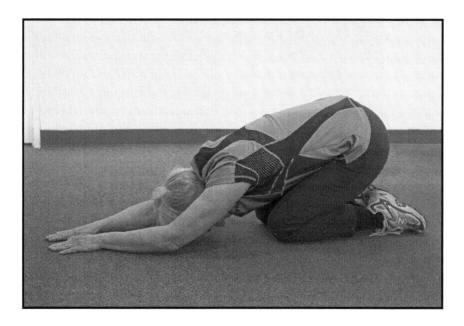

The Bow—Back, Shoulders, Arms Stretch

Kneel on a firm surface. Fold your body down with your arms extended forward near your head.

Gradually walk your fingers out until your arms and body feel elongated.

Relax into this stretch and feel the tension leaving your body. If you are more flexible, you may be able to "sit on your feet" while in the full elongated stretch.

Hold 30 to 60 seconds.

In all of these stretches be sure to consciously take note of your breathing. Exhale as you go into the stretch. Then keep breathing deeply in a rhythmical manner as you hold the stretch.

ABOUT THE AUTHORS

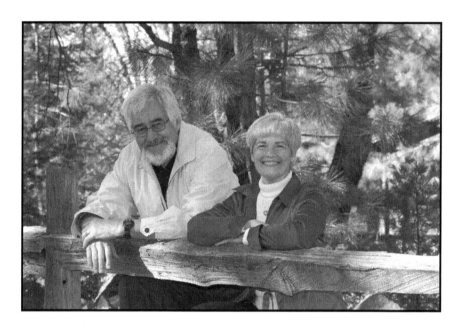

Pat and Jo Tillman, a team for over 50 years, married in 1964 and attended professional school together. Pat graduated from Golden Gate College of Law and Jo from the University of California Medical School, San Francisco in 1970. After passing the bar exam and finishing internship they moved to northern California where they practiced for many years.

Besides his legal practice Pat helped establish Emergency Medical Services, pre-hospital care, in rural northern California and volunteered as an emergency medical technician. Dr. Jo was one of the first full time emergency room physicians in this area throughout the 1970's.

She then switched from "putting out" the fires, to preventing the fires of ill health and degenerative disease, opening her "Wellness" clinic in 1983. From that time to now she has pursued a quest to discover the underlying causes of disease instead of primarily treating the symptoms. She was a pioneer. Thankfully now many physicians are looking at and teaching about those underlying causes of disease: poor nutrition, lack of exercise and toxicity.

In their family Dr. Jo became the expert on nutrition and Pat led the way in exercise. And now they combine their expertise and experience to present *Fit in 15* to you, the best of exercise and nutrition.

REFERENCES

Chapter 1

[1] Mayo Clin Proc. Jun 2012; 87(6): 587-595.doi: 10.1016/j.mayocp.2012.04.005 PMCID: PMC3538475 Potential Adverse Cardiovascular Effects From Excessive Endurance Exercise James H. O'Keefe,a,[low asterisk] Harshal R. Patil,a Carl J. Lavie,b Anthony Magalski,a Robert A. Vogel,c and Peter A. McCulloughd

http://www.ncbi.nlm.nih.gov/pmc/articles/PMC3538475/

[2] Europeans Heart Journal, Risk of arrhythmias in 52 755 long-distance cross-country skiers: a cohort study Kasper Andersen, Bahman Farahmand, Anders Ahlbom, Claes Held, Sverker Ljunghall, Karl Michaëlsson, Johan Sundström DOI: http://dx.doi.org/10.1093/eurheartj/eht188 First published online: 11 June 2013 http://eurheartj.oxfordjournals.org/content/early/2013/06/10/eurheartj.eht188.full

[3] http://delfinovi.com/reading/brief-history-of-slow-motion-training-serious-strength-VQEe.html

[4] http://news.google.com/newspapers?nid=1964&dat=19880802&id=g9BVAAAAIBAJ&sjid=xkANAAAAIBAJ&pg=2014,900620&hl=en Newspaper article from the Palm Beach Post August 2, 1988

Chapter 2 No End Notes

Chapter 3

[5] http://www.sszrc.com/articles/What_is_SuperSlow.pdf by Ken Hutchins, Owner of Trade mark SuperSlow

[6] http://news.google.com/newspapers?nid=1964&dat=19880802&id=g9BVAAAAIBAJ&sjid=xkANAAAAIBAJ&pg=2014,900620&hl=en Newspaper article from the Palm Beach Post August 2, 1988

Chapter 4

[7] Prevalence and Trends of Metabolic Syndrome in the Adult U.S. Population, 1999-2010. Hiram Beltrán-Sánchez, PhD*; Michael O. Harhay, MPH†; Meera M. Harhay, MD‡; Sean McElligott, MS†

J Am Coll Cardiol. 2013;62(8):697-703. doi:10.1016/j.jacc.2013.05.064 http://content.onlinejacc.org/article.aspx?articleid=1709463

[8] http://circ.ahajournals.org/content/118/4/346.short

[9] http://www.ncbi.nlm.nih.gov/pubmed/12797841 Sports Med. 2003;33(8):599-613. The exercise-induced growth hormone response in athletes. Godfrey RJ1, Madgwick Z, Whyte GP

[10] Harper's Review of Biochemistry, 18th edition, page 506.

[11] http://www.optimalhealthpartner.com/A_Archive/Growth%20 Hormone/Albert_LoDose%20GH%20and%20Obesity.pdf Albert SG, Mooradian AD. J Clin Endocrinol Metab. 2004 Feb;89(2):695-701.

[12] http://press.endocrine.org/doi/abs/10.1210/jcem.75.1.1619005

[13] http://link.springer.com/article/10.1007/s00421-001-0568-y#page-1

[14] https://news.google.com/newspapers?nid=1964&dat=19880802&id= g9BVAAAAIBAJ&sjid=xkANAAAAIBAJ&pg=2014,900620&hl=en Newspaper article from the Palm Beach Post August 2, 1988

[15] http://www.nature.com/ijo/journal/v32/n4/abs/0803781a.html

[16] Aging in motion: the facts about sarcopenia. Alliance for Aging Research website. http://www.aginginmotion.org/wp-content/ uploads/2011/04/sarcopenia_fact_sheet.pdf. Updated April 2011. Accessed March 19, 2012.

[17] http://www.ncbi.nlm.nih.gov/pubmed/21396499 Am J Med. 2011 Mar;124(3):194-8. doi: 10.1016/j.amjmed.2010.08.020. Resistance exercise for the aging adult: clinical implications and prescription guidelines. Peterson MD1, Gordon PM.

[18] *Body by Science*, Doug McGuff and John Little, McGraw-Hill books, © 2009.

[19] http://circ.ahajournals.org/content/101/7/828/T1.expansion.html

[20] http://www.cdc.gov/pcd/issues/2014/14_0007.htm

[21] Dr. Mercola interviews Dr. McGuff: http://fitness.mercola.com/sites/ fitness/archive/2012/01/06/dr-doug-mcguff-on-exercise.aspx

[22] http://circ.ahajournals.org/content/118/4/346.short

[23] http://www.mayoclinic.org/diseases-conditions/high-blood- pressure/expert-answers/weightlifting/faq-20058451

[24] http://www.webmd.com/fitness-exercise/features/lift-slow-to-get-fit- fast SuperSlow increases HDL cholesterol

[25] http://www.sciencedirect.com/science/article/pii/S0278691513003529 Food and Chemical Toxicology Volume 61, November 2013, Pages 171-177 Mechanisms involved in oxidative stress regulation

[26] http://physther.org/content/91/6/894.full Journal of the American Physical Therapy Association

[27] http://www.ncbi.nlm.nih.gov/pubmed/16506871 Phys Ther. 2006 Mar;86(3):345-54.

[28] https://krex.k-state.edu/dspace/bitstream/handle/2097/4133/CaliDunham2010.pdf?sequence=9 THE EFFECTS OF HIGH INTENSITY INTERVAL TRAINING ON PULMONARY FUNCTION By CALI A DUNHAM B.S., Kansas State University, 2008

[29] http://www.amednews.com/article/20080915/health/309159977/4/

[30] http://www.amenclinics.com/

[31] http://www.ncbi.nlm.nih.gov/pubmed/21817111 J Appl Physiol (1985). 2011 Oct;111(4):1066-71. doi: 10.1152/japplphysiol.00343.2011. Epub 2011 Aug 4. Exercise training increases mitochondrial biogenesis in the brain. Steiner JL1, Murphy EA, McClellan JL, Carmichael MD, Davis JM.

[32] http://www.ncbi.nlm.nih.gov/pubmed/18595904 BMJ. 2008 Jul 1;337:a439. doi: 10.1136/bmj.a439. Association between muscular strength and mortality in men: prospective cohort study.

[33] http://www.greenmedinfo.com/article/exercise-training-can-help-minimize-detrimental-skeletal-muscle-aging-deficits Am J Physiol Regul Integr Comp Physiol. 2012 May 9. Epub 2012 May 9. PMID: 22573103

[34] http://www.greenmedinfo.com/blog/exercise-stops-mitochondrial-aging-process-its-tracks

[35] http://www.ncbi.nlm.nih.gov/pubmed/12797841 Sports Med. 2003;33(8):599-613. The exercise-induced growth hormone response in athletes. Godfrey RJ1, Madgwick Z, Whyte GP

Chapter 5

[36] Dr. Mercola interviews Dr. McGuff: http://fitness.mercola.com/sites/fitness/archive/2012/01/06/dr-doug-mcguff-on-exercise.aspx

[37] http://ajcn.nutrition.org/content/62/1/1.short Am J Clin Nutr July 1995 vol. 62 no. 1 1-9

[38] http://ajp.psychiatryonline.org/doi/abs/10.1176/ajp.152.3.419 Am J of Psychiatry Volume 152 Issue 3, March 1995, pp. 419-423

[39] http://journals.lww.com/epidem/Abstract/2001/03000/Low_Serum_Cholesterol_Concentration_and_Risk_of.7.aspx Epidemiology:March 2001 - Volume 12 - Issue 2 - pp 168-172

[40] http://articles.mercola.com/sites/articles/archive/2014/12/31/bitter-truth-sugar.aspx?e_cid=20141231Z1-USCanada_DNL_art_1&utm_source=dnl&utm_medium=email&utm_content=art1&utm_campaign=20141231Z1-USCanada&et_cid=DM63348&et_rid=787042024

[41] http://www.pnas.org/content/111/47/16647.abstract Proceedings of the National Academy of Sciences November 25, 2014: 111(47); 16647-16653

[42] Intermountain Medical Center, Eurekalert April 3, 2011 http://www.eurekalert.org/pub_releases/2011-04/imc-sfr033111.php

[43] American Journal of Clinical Nutrition November 2009: 90(5); 1138-1143 http://ajcn.nutrition.org/content/90/5/1138.short

[44] International Journal of Obesity May 2011: 35, 714-727 http://www.nature.com/ijo/journal/v35/n5/full/ijo2010171a.html

[45] http://fitness.mercola.com/sites/fitness/archive/2015/01/30/time-restricted-eating.aspx?e_cid=20150130Z1_DNL_RTL_B_art_1&utm_source=dnl&utm_medium=email&utm_content=art1&utm_campaign=20150130Z1_RTL_B&et_cid=DM68176&et_rid=824589341

[46] Nutrition & Metabolism May 17, 2012 http://www.nutritionandmetabolism.com/content/pdf/1743-7075-9-40.pdf

[47] Medicine & Science in Sports & Exercise May 2010 - Volume 42 - Issue 5 - pp 998-1003 http://journals.lww.com/acsm-msse/Abstract/2010/05000/Timing_Protein_Intake_Increases_Energy_Expenditure.21.aspx

[48] http://fitness.mercola.com/sites/fitness/archive/2013/02/01/whey-protein-improves-hgh.aspx

[49] http://fitness.mercola.com/sites/fitness/archive/2011/05/11/whey-protein-shown-superior-to-other-milk-proteins-for-building-muscle.aspx

Chapter 6

[50] https://www.acsm.org/docs/brochures/high-intensity-interval-training.pdf

[51] http://fitness.mercola.com/sites/fitness/archive/2012/02/10/phil-campbell-interview.aspx

Pat and Dr. Jo Tillman

[52] http://en.wikipedia.org/wiki/High-intensity_interval_training

[53] https://www.acsm.org/docs/brochures/high-intensity-interval-training.pdf

[54] http://jap.physiology.org/content/98/6/1983

[55] http://www.budopoint.de/en/science/articles/IntenseTraining.pdf Journal of Applied Physiology 2005; 98: 1985-1990

[56] http://www.wou.edu/~kiddk/PE%20359/2013_Handbook/Risk_Management/ViewandRead/HighIntensityTraining.pdf

[57] http://www.ncbi.nlm.nih.gov/pubmed/11772161 Sports Med. 2002;32(1):53-73. The scientific basis for high-intensity interval training: optimising training programmes and maximising performance in highly trained endurance athletes. Laursen PB1, Jenkins DG.

Chapter 7

[58] http://www.amazon.com/Move-Little-Lose-Lot-N-E-A-T/dp/B005ZOFWTU

[59] BMJ January 21, 2015 http://blogs.bmj.com/bjsm/2015/01/21/sitting-ducks-sedentary-behaviour-and-its-health-risks-part-one-of-a-two-part-series/

[60] http://www.gruvetechnologies.com/neat.html

[61] http://www.beyondhealthnews.com/wpnews/index.php/2014/02/the-hazards-of-sitting/

[62] http://www.latimes.com/science/sciencenow/la-sci-sn-get-up-20140731-story.html

[63] Stretching: Bob Anderson; Shelter Publications, Inc. © 1980 http://www.sharecare.com/health/flexibility-training/long-should-hold-a-stretch http://www.stretching-exercises-guide.com/how-long-to-stretch.html http://www.drillsandskills.com/article/11 http://www.sportsscience.co/flexibility/how-often-and-how-long-should-i-stretch-to-improve-flexibility/

INDEX